# How to Good-bye Depression

## Hiroyuki Nishigaki

Writers Club Press

San Jose  New York  Lincoln  Shanghai

**How to Good-bye Depression**

Published by Writers Club Press
an imprint of iUniverse.com, Inc.

For information address:
iUniverse.com, Inc.
5220 S 16th, Ste. 200
Lincoln, NE 68512
www.iuniverse.com

ISBN: 0-595-09472-4

Printed in the United States of America

# Contents

# Part 1 If you constrict anus 100 times everyday

I think it is effective to cure or prevent depression and become happy-healthy-efficient that you (1)constrict anus 100 times in succession and dent navel 100 times in succession after constricting anus 100 times in succession everyday following the life style of long-lived British as possible (2)sometimes turn to bay throwing away pride-welcome a insult or fall into the hell voluntarily or occupy your time with something else (anything would do) (3) enjoy taking advantage of a petty tyrant to temper yourself (4)do 3-week fasting and excrete a bucketful of old black solid excrement which has stuck to your small intestine for long years (5)reduce the frequency of sex or masturbation to less than half if possible (6)rotate your energetic vortex of your body.

Subject:    Re: How to good-by depression
From:       pjl
Date:       1999/12/13
Message-ID:
Newsgroups:

Hiroyuki Nishigaki wrote:

> Hello
> How to good-by depression is how to strengthen your internal organ and how to grow younger. I think it is effective to

constrict your anus 100 times in succession and dent your navel100 times in succession everyday.

Hiroyuki Nishigaki Spirit bless you!

yes, good-by as i pick myself off the floor still laughing.

thank-you my friend.

Opet

Subject:    How to good-by depression 1
From:       Hiroyuki Nishigaki
Date:       1999/12/13
Message-ID:
Newsgroups: depression

Hello

How to good-by depression is how to strengthen your internal organs, how to have good complexion and how to grow younger. I think it is effective to constrict your anus 100 times, dent your navel 100 times in succession everyday. You can do so at a boring meeting or in a subway without being noticed for you to do so. I have known 70 year old man who has practiced it for 20 years. As a result, he has good complexion and has grown 20 years younger. His eyes sparkle. He is full of vigor, happiness, and joy. He has neither complained nor born a grudge under any circumstance.

Furthermore, he can make ** three times in succession without drawing out.

Sincerely.

Hiroyuki Nishigaki

Spirit bless you!

Subject:   Re: How to good-by depression 1
From:      Rsh
Date:      1999/12/13
Message-ID:
Newsgroups: depression
[More Headers]

> Shit, what is this gobbledygook?
> WHAT did he make three times in succession????
> I GOTTA KNOW NOW!!!!!!!!
> Aawa, in suspense

Constrict your anus 100 times, and the answer will be revealed to you.


Subject:   Re: How to good-by depression 1
From:      Aawa
Date:      1999/12/13
Message-ID:
Newsgroups: depression
[More Headers]

On 13 Dec 1999 15:11:57 GMT, Hiroyuki Nishigaki wrote:

> Furthermore, he can make ** three times in succession
> without drawing out.
> Shit, what is this gobbledygook?
> WHAT did he make three times in succession????
> I GOTTA KNOW NOW!!!!!!!!
> Aawa, in suspense

—Toto…I don't think we're in Kansas anymore.

Subject:    Re: How to good-by depression 1
From:        Rse
Date:        1999/12/13
Message-ID:
Newsgroups: depression
[More Headers]

Hiroyuki Nishigaki wrote:

> Hello for 20 years. As a result, he has good complexion and
> has grown 20 years younger.

So, he started when he was 50, and he grew 20 years
younger during those 20 years, so he must still be 50, but you
say he's 70, so he must really be 90, which would make him
70. No, wait, he's grown 20 years younger. Then 20 years ago,
he was 110? Um, can I see this guy's birth certificate? I'm getting really confused here.

—Rse

Subject:    Re: How to good-by depression 1
From:        Rse
Date:        1999/12/18
Message-ID:
Newsgroups: depression
[More Headers]

And then Mistress Hiroyuki Nishigaki didst E-Mail the "official
mineral of the millenium" with all square box characters included:

Hello

He is 70 years old, but looks like 50 years old. I have practiced so almost everyday for about 18 years, too after I was
taught to practice so by him. As a result, I looks like 38-48

years old although I am 58 years old. I owe much gratitude to him now. I hope you will practice so. It will pay you well. You will begin to have better complexion, grow younger and have happy lucky feeling little by little. I recommend you will take one hour stroll everyday, too if possible. You had better co?strict your anus 100 times in succession everyday at least.

Sincerely.
Hiroyuki Nishigaki

Hiroyuki Nishigaki wrote in article

Hello

How to good-by depression is how to strengthen your internal organ and how to grow younger. I think it is effective to constrict your anus 100 times in succession and dent your navel100 times in succession everyday.


Subject:    Re: How to good-by depression
From:       Stb
Date:       1999/12/14
Message-ID:
Newsgroups: depression
[More Headers]

Thank you Hiroyuki. I will certainly have to try this and see how quickly it will cure my depression.

—Stb
Montreal, Canada

Subject:    Re: How to good-by depression
From:       Bcof
Date:       999/12/13
Message-ID:
Newsgroups:
[More Headers]

Hmmmm guess this wont for me....too much lint in my navel.

CJ wont say how anal this post is!


Subject:    Re: How to good-by depression
From:       brss
Date:       1999/12/13
Message-ID:
Newsgroups:
[More Headers]

I once dented my anus in the Navy. I was put on constrictive duty.

This happened 100 times. Bahahaha!


Subject:    Re: How to good-by depression
From:       Aawa
Date:       1999/12/13
Message-ID:
Newsgroups: depression
[More Headers]

On 13 Dec 1999 14:40:14 GMT, Hiroyuki Nishigaki wrote:

Hello

How to good-by depression is how to strengthen your internal organ and how to grow younger. I think it is effective to constrict your anus 100 times in succession and dent your navel100 times in succession everyday.

Hiroyuki Nishigaki
Spirit bless you!

I'm SO glad I didn't have coffee in my mouth when I read this!!!
ROTFLMAO!!!!!!!!!!

Aawa

—Toto…I don't think we're in Kansas anymore.


Subject:   Re: How to good-by depression
From:     Cdis
Date:     1999/12/13
Message-ID:
Newsgroups: depression
[More Headers]

Hiroyuki Nishigaki wrote in message

Hello

How to good-by depression is how to strengthen your internal organ and how to grow younger. I think it is effective to constrict your anus 100 times in succession and dent your navel100 times in succession everyday.

Hiroyuki Nishigaki
Spirit bless you!

This is priceless. You just can't buy this sort of thing. This gets forwarded to my friends.

Subject:    Re: How to good-by depression
From:       Xyuk
Date:       1999/12/17
Message-ID:
Newsgroups: depression

Mary Frances wrote:

By the way, how do I get to Libra?
I'm not sure you want to. We're strange folks.
Mary, who has the sun, Venus, & Uranus (& hers, as well) in Libra
So, then…you're a Libra-rian? And, where is Myanus?

Subject:    Re: How to good-by depression
From:       Jll
Date:       1999/12/16
Message-ID:
Newsgroups: depression
[More Headers]

'Splenetic' means testy, not tastey ·unless, of course, you like that sort of thing.

Jll

Subject:    Re: How to good-by depression
From:       Xyuk
Date:       1999/12/21
Message-ID: 385FDC3C.CDDEDF97@writeme.com
Newsgroups: depression
[More Headers]

   Is there an anal constriction video and half-hour info-mercial?


Subject:    Re: How to good-by depression
From:       Bcs
Date:       1999/12/19
Message-ID:
Newsgroups: depression

   i just want to let everyone know that i have been able to good-
bye depression totally without benefit of anal constriction!
   I certainly hope so…that's a ghastly thought. No doubt an
example of "retaining your way out of depression" :)

                                                        Tae


Subject:    Re: How to good-by depression
From:       Xyuk
Date:       1999/12/17
Message-ID:
Newsgroups: depression

Aawa wrote:

   x-no-archive: yes
   posted only

So, then…you're a Libra-rian? And, where is Myanus?
I got Uranus right here, buddy…
LOL
Guy
I have the Uranus wav if anyone wants it.

Aawa

This I gotta see…Uranus wav….
(talk about letting it all hang out!)


Subject:    Re: How to good-by depression
From:       Xyuk
Date:        1999/12/14
Message-ID:
Newsgroups: depression
[More Headers]

Alan Harding wrote: In article, Hiroyuki Nishigaki writes

Hello
How to good-by depression is how to strengthen your internal organ and how to grow younger.
I have no intention of doing anything so unNatural as growing younger!
I might try strengthening my internal organ tho….

Subject:    Re: How to good-by depression
From:       Dff
Date:       1999/12/14
Message-ID:
Newsgroups: depression
[More Headers]

On 13 Dec 1999 14:40:14 GMT, Hiroyuki Nishigaki wrote:

Hello

How to good-by depression is how to strengthen your internal organ and how to grow younger. I think it is effective to constrict your anus 100 times in succession and dent your navel100 times in succession everyday.

> Hiroyuki Nishigaki
> Spirit bless you!

may the belly-button lint goddesses preserve and protect your fuzziness for all of the rest of your days.

Subject:    Re: How to good-by depression
From:       Rsh
Date:       1999/12/14
Message-ID:
Newsgroups: depression
[More Headers]

Dent! Constrict! Dent! Constrict! Dent! Constrict! Dent! Constrict! Dent!

Constrict! Dent! Constrict! Dent! Constrict! Dent! Constrict! Dent!

Constrict! Dent! Constrict! Dent! Constrict! Dent! Constrict! Dent!

Constrict! Dent! Constrict! Dent! Constrict! Dent! Constrict! Dent!

Constrict! Dent! Constrict! Dent! Constrict! Dent! Constrict!

Subject:    Re: How to good-by depression
From:       Lmf
Date:       1999/12/14
Message-ID:
Newsgroups: depression
[More Headers]

In article, Xyuk wrote:

AB wrote: I once dented my anus in the Navy. I was put on constrictive duty. This happened 100 times. Bahahaha!

I though your anus was a planet....

My anus is in Libra. So is Uranus.

Lmf

* Sent from RQ http://www.rq.com The Internet's Discussion Network *

The fastest and easiest way to search and participate in Usenet-Free!

Subject:    Re: How to good-by depression
From:       Cbok
Date:       1999/12/13
Message-ID:
Newsgroups: depression

I think it is effective to constrict your anus 100 times in succession

Welllllllllllllllll…first you'd need to remove your head from there.

Ijam

Say it out loud. I'm depressed and I'm proud. well….just depressed

OWWWW!!!!!! I don't feel good…

In a funk but always funky, and with plenty of soul.

Subject:    Re: How to good-by depression
From:        Abee
Date:        1999/12/13
Message-ID:
Newsgroups: depression
[More Headers]

Cdis wrote: Hiroyuki Nishigaki wrote in message news:

Hello

How to good-by depression is how to strengthen your internal organ and how to grow younger. I think it is effective to constrict your anus 100 times in succession and dent your navel100 times in succession everyday.

Hiroyuki Nishigaki<br>Spirit bless you!

This is priceless. You just can't buy this sort of thing. This gets forwarded to my friends.

Ok, it is established that I am a tech slow. But is the price-lessness the post in asd or the homepage I just checked out?

Bryce

constricting his mind so far

Subject:    Re: How to good-by depression
From:       Xyuk
Date:       1999/12/13
Message-ID:
Newsgroups: depression
[More Headers]

Ab wrote:

I once dented my anus in the Navy. I was put on constric-tive duty.

This happened 100 times. Bahahaha!

I though your anus was a planet….

Subject:    Re: How to good-by depression
From:       Jlud
Date:       1999/12/13
Message-ID:
Newsgroups: depression
[More Headers]

this seems like something that would be on the Radiohead website.

i try to constrict my anus at least ten times a day and i don't feel much better…

—Dedw

Musician Search Online

Jlud

Bdis wrote in message news:
Hiroyuki Nishigaki wrote in message news:

Hello

How to good-by depression is how to strengthen your internal organ and how to grow younger. I think it is effective to constrict your anus 100 times in succession and dent your navel100 times in succession everyday.

Hiroyuki Nishigaki
Spirit bless you!

This is priceless. You just can't buy this sort of thing. This gets forwarded to my friends.


Subject:   Re: How to good-by depression
From:      Jll
Date:      1999/12/16
Message-ID:
Newsgroups: depression
[More Headers]

'Splenetic' means testy, not tastey ·unless, of course, you like that sort of thing.

Jll

Subject:    Re: How to good-by depression
From:       Xyuk
Date:        1999/12/16
Message-ID:
Newsgroups: depression
[More Headers]

Jll wrote:

'Splenetic' means testy, not tastey ·unless, of course, you like that sort of thing.
Are men, then, bi-splenetic?


Subject:    RE: How to good-by depression
From:       Lms
Date:        1999/12/16
Message-ID:
Newsgroups: depression
[More Headers]

Anal bullworker? Sounds like a tough job! But I guess you gotta keep the bulls happy.

—Lms


Subject:    Re: How to good-by depression
From:       Aawa
Date:        1999/12/16
Message-ID:
Newsgroups: depression
[More Headers]

On Thu, 16 Dec 1999 16:13:58 GMT, Lms wrote:

Anal bullworker? Sounds like a tough job! But I guess you gotta keep the bulls happy.
Isn't that a rural type thingie?
No, wait-that was sheep.
Nevermind.

Aawa

—Toto…I don't think we're in Kansas anymore.


Subject:    Re: How to good-by depression
From:      Bcar
Date:      1999/12/14
Message-ID:
Newsgroups: depression

I haven't laughed this hard in years. We need a lot more anus constricting posts!
\* Sent from RQ http://www.rq.com The Internet's Discussion Network \*
The fastest and easiest way to search and participate in Usenet-Free!


Subject:    Re: How to good-by depression
From:      Hiroyuki Nishigaki
Date:      1999/12/14
Message-ID:
Newsgroups: depression

Hello

I have read your contribution with pleasure Just now. The spirit bless you. Furthermore, I recommend you take one-hour stroll everyday if possible.

Hiroyuki Nishigaki
Spirit bless you!


Subject:    Re: How to good-by depression
From:      Abea
Date:       1999/12/14
Message-ID:
Newsgroups: depression

Hiroyuki-

I have been trying your technique, and I am sorry to say that it has not had any effect on my depression. I am now able, though, to crack walnuts with my buttocks. Do you know of any practical application for this ability, or any job prospects in the Nut Industry?

Thank you.

—

```
               ‾
   Abea     _.-’ )
        (_. ‘\__
         \_ ^/ _)
        .-’_   \
       (_.’\    ‘—.
        /_ ſ -._/
         (_/
```

Subject:   Re: How to good-by depression
From:      Hie
Date:      1999/12/17
Message-ID:
Newsgroups: depression

please, everyone, don't be fooled into attempting this method!
(although i've heard that it can have limited success if done
under strict medical supervision) i just want to let everyone
know that i have been able to good-bye depression totally without benefit of anal constriction! it's true, i swear! well, okay,
maybe i did dent my navel a few times...but not anywhere near
100! my navel, by the way is also in gemini, but i haven't seen
doug's anus at all! and i've been looking for it! rat.

                                                                    mad

ps my spellcheck always wants to change 'doug' to
'dough'...maybe he's rich? or really bakes well?
"And yes I said yes I will Yes."

                                                                   -Hie-


Subject:   Re: How to good-by depression
From:      Lmf
Date:      1999/12/16

In article, Xyuk wrote:

My anus is a Gemini...which is not to be confused with 'e
pluribus anum'.... and not on every coin of the realm....
By the way, how do I get to Libra?
I'm not sure you want to. We're strange folks.

Mary, who has the sun, Venus, & Uranus (& hers, as well) in Libra

* Sent from RQ http://www.rq.com The Internet's Discussion Network *

The fastest and easiest way to search and participate in Usenet-Free!

Subject:    Re: How to good-by depression
From:       Xyuk
Date:       1999/12/15
Message-ID:
Newsgroups: depression

Lmf wrote:

In article, Xyuk wrote:

AB wrote:

I once dented my anus in the Navy. I was put on constrictive duty.

This happened 100 times. Bahahaha!

I though your anus was a planet….

My anus is in Libra. So is Uranus.

Lmf

My anus is a Gemini…which is not to be confused with 'e pluribus anum'…. and not on every coin of the realm….

By the way, how do I get to Libra?

Cdou

Subject:   Re: How to good-by depression
From:      Aah
Date:      1999/12/14
Message-ID:
Newsgroups: depression

In article, Xyuk writes

Aah wrote:
In article, Hiroyuki Nishigaki writes
How to good-by depression is how to strengthen your internal organ and how to grow younger.

I have no intention of doing anything so unNatural as growing younger!

I might try strengthening my internal organ tho....

Did you have any particular organ in mind? I'm a sucker for the first book I see on how to strengthen my spleen. I have no idea what it does, but having a stronger one would surely allow me to use the splendid word 'splenetic' much more often, which must be a Good Thing, mustn't it?

          —Aah

~~~~~~~~~~~

The opinions given above may be mine. They might also just be what I feel like saying right now, okay?

Subject:   Re: i got my navel pierced.
From:      Rse
Date:      1999/12/15
Message-ID:
Newsgroups: depression
[More Headers]

but now how can you do mistress Hiroyuki Nishigaki's belly button squeezing exercises to "good-by depression"? :)

—Rse

Subject:    Re: How to good-by depression
From:       Aah
Date:       1999/12/16
Message-ID:
Newsgroups: depression
[More Headers]

In article, Iju writes

On Tue, 14 Dec 1999 22:00:09 +0000, AAH wrote:

In article, Xyuk writes

Aah wrote:

In article, Hiroyuki Nishigaki writes

How to good-by depression is how to strengthen your internal organ and how to grow younger.

I have no intention of doing anything so unNatural as growing younger!

I might try strengthening my internal organ tho....

Did you have any particular organ in mind? I'm a sucker for the first book I see on how to strengthen my spleen. I have no idea what it does, but having a stronger one would surely allow me to use the splendid word 'splenetic' much more often, which must be a Good Thing, mustn't it?

Oh goody :) "splenetic". more word food.

Ummm...errr...so what does it mean? :)

In the same way that renal means 'of the kidneys', and cardiac means 'of the heart', you'd expect celeriac to mean 'of the spleen', wouldn't you?

Well it doesn't, but splenetic does.

In the same way that the heart is, as everyone knows, the seat of certain emotions, so is the spleen. Splenetic means bad-tempered, irritable and/or melancholy. Not a word likely to be much used in these parts, surely, but people might know someone at work or home they can safely use it about. Quite probably even in their hearing.

Iju (whose stupid little pocket dictionary doesn't help at all!)

I love dictionaries. If ever the price of the Oxford Dictionary CD set comes down, I shall get an extra CD-drive to keep it permanently in. I suppose it might already have come down, I haven't checked the price for, oh, days. Something to do today. :)

—Aah

~~~~~~~~~~~~~~~~~~~~~~~~~~~~~~~~~~~~~~~~~~~~~~~~
~~~~~~~~~~~~~~~~~~~~~~~~~~~~~

The opinions given above may be mine. They might also just be what I feel like saying right now, okay?


Subject:    How to good-by depression 2
From:       Hiroyuki Nishigaki
Date:       1999/12/16
Message-ID:
Newsgroups: depression
[More Headers]

Hello

I have also constricted my anus and dented my navel 100 times in succession almost everyday for about 18 years after I was taught by him. As a result, I have grown 10-20 years younger. Furthermore, I can overcome the stress of various complains which are the causes of depression. I owe much gratitude to him now.

I recommend you will take one hour stroll everyday, too if possible.

Hiroyuki Nishigaki
Spirit bless you!

Subject:    Re: How to good-by depression 2
From:       Kls
Date:       1999/12/19
Message-ID:
Newsgroups: depression
[More Headers]

In article, Dfb writes

The only way your anus can lift barbells is if you have some very strong hemerroids.

ROFL! thank you! I needed to laugh, and you just cracked me up!

—Kls

"damaged people are dangerous, they know they can survive"

Subject:    Re: How to good-by depression 2
From:       Rsh
Date:       1999/12/17
Message-ID:
Newsgroups: depression
[More Headers]

But what would an anus-constrictor be like? And just how *would* my overly-young trainer teach me, an old woman in his mind, to use it??

Yeah, baby, I see a HUGE market here! The Blues-Be-Gone (R) Anus Constrictor by Ronco. Late night infomercials... celebrity endorsements (William Shatner, Suzanne Sommers, Bob Hope?).... sweepstakes!

the whole works.

yeah...I can see it now...


Subject:   Re: How to good-by depression 2
From:      Aawa
Date:      1999/12/16
Message-ID:
Newsgroups: depression
[More Headers]

On Thu, 16 Dec 1999 10:37:30-0000, Cdis wrote:

How old were you, and how old are you now?

I'm intrigued...just how do you constrict the anus? Is it like trying to hold it in when you desperately need to do a poo? Or does it involve the use of some kind of anal bull-worker or dumbells?

Anal dumbells?

I've met a few of those before!

Aawa

—Toto...I don't think we're in Kansas anymore.

Subject:    Re: How to good-by depression 2
From:       Dfb
Date:       1999/12/16
Message-ID:
Newsgroups: depression
[More Headers]

The only way your anus can lift barbells is if you have some very strong hemerroids.

* Sent from RQ http://www.rq.com The Internet's Discussion Network *

The fastest and easiest way to search and participate in Usenet-Free!


Subject:    Re: How to good-by depression 2
From:       Abok
Date:       1999/12/15
Message-ID:
Newsgroups: depression
[More Headers]

Hiroyuki Nishigaki wrote:

I recommend you will take one hour stroll everyday, too if possible.

I recommend you take a hike.

Spirit bless you. ;-)

Ijam

—"Once you become aware of this force for unity in life, you can't ever forget it.

It becomes part of everything you do."

—JC 'Meditations'
Visit The Abok Cafe
http://www.geocities.com/SoHo/Study/

Subject:   Re: How to good-by depression 2
From:     Yzoe
Date:     1999/12/16
Message-ID:
Newsgroups: depression
[More Headers]

huh?

On 16 Dec 1999 05:19:24 GMT, Hiroyuki Nishigaki wrote:

Hello

I have also constricted my anus and dented my navel 100 times in succession almost everyday for about 18 years after I was taught by him. As a result, I have grown 10-20 years younger. Furthermore, I can overcome the stress of various complains which are the causes of depression. I owe much gratitude to him now.

I recommend you will take one hour stroll everyday, too if possible.

Hiroyuki Nishigaki
Spirit bless you!

Subject:    Re: How to good-by depression 2
From:       Hiroyuki Nishigaki
Date:       1999/12/18
Message-ID:
Newsgroups: depression
[More Headers]

Dear Yzoe

Huh? I recommend you challenge. You will never wonder huh? after you practice so for a few months. A female Yoga teacher is my first person that I taught to do so 17 years ago. When I taught her, she was sad and lonely very much because of her husband death. She has no children. She has practiced so everyday for 17 years after I taught her. She says thank you and give a present to me whenever I meet her. She say "By the grace of your teaching, I can live happily and vigorously without my husband although I am 80 years old".

Hiroyuki Nishigaki
Spirit bless you!

Subject:    Re: How to good-by depression 2
From:       Aawa
Date:       1999/12/18
Message-ID:
Newsgroups: depression
[More Headers]

On 18 Dec 1999 15:01:13 GMT, Hiroyuki Nishigaki wrote:

Dear Yzoe

Huh? I recommend you challenge. You will never wonder huh? after you practice so for a few months. A female Yoga teacher is my first person that I taught to do so 17 years ago. When I taught her, she was sad and lonely very much because of her husband death. She has no children. She has practiced so everyday for 17 years after I taught her. She says thank you and give a present to me whenever I meet her. She say "By the grace of your teaching, I can live happily and vigorously without my husband although I am 80 years old".

Hiroyuki Nishigaki

Spirit bless you!
Yea? What kind of er, present-?
Aawa, imagining
—Toto…I don't think we're in Kansas anymore.


Subject:    Re: How to good-by depression 2
From:       Cdis
Date:       1999/12/16
Message-ID:
Newsgroups: depression
[More Headers]

Hiroyuki Nishigaki wrote in message news:

Hello

I have also constricted my anus and dented my navel 100 times in succession almost everyday for about 18 years after I was taught by him. As a result, I have grown 10-20 years younger. Furthermore, I can overcome the stress of various complains which are the causes of depression. I owe much gratitude to him now.

How old were you, and how old are you now?

I'm intrigued…just how do you constrict the anus? Is it like trying to hold it in when you desperately need to do a poo? Or does it involve the use of some kind of anal bull-worker or dumbells?

Subject:    To constrict anus is Yoga way, too
From:       Hiroyuki Nishigaki
Date:       1999/12/18
Message-ID:
Newsgroups: depression
[More Headers]

Dear, sir

To constrict anus 100 times in succession and dent navel 100 times in succession after constricting anus is very simple. It is one of the secret ways of Yoga to strengthen body and heart, too. You do not need any implement. If you do so every-day, you will learn the trick soon. I think you will begin to have peculiar happy lucky feeling in a month or a few months little by little.

I have received the present today, too which one who has practiced it for a year sent to me. If you practice it, confirm the effect and teach it to someone, someone will owe much grati-tude to you. If we can give joy to someone at first, someone will give joy to us. I think it is a good medicine to prevent or cure depression.

Hiroyuki Nishigaki
Spirit bless you!

Subject:    Re: To constrict anus is Yoga way, too
From:       Fgro
Date:       1999/12/18
Newsgroups: depression
[More Headers]

okay, so it might give you good abs, but who wants to be a tight ass?

just a thought.

Bcar

Subject:    Re: To constrict anus is Yoga way, too
From:       Opan
Date:       1999/12/18
Newsgroups: depression
[More Headers]

On 18 Dec 1999 06:41:43 GMT, Fgro wrote:

okay, so it might give you good abs, but who wants to be a tight ass?

just a thought.

Bcar
Prof

Subject:    Re: To constrict anus is Yoga way, too
From:       Lms
Date:       1999/12/18
Newsgroups: depression
[More Headers]

On 18 Dec 1999 06 :22:38 GMT, Hiroyuki Nishigaki wrote:

Dear, sir
some snipped stuff
I think you will begin to have peculiar happy lucky feeling
in a month or a few months little by little.
oh, I have a peculiar feeling, alright.

Lms

Subject:   Re: To constrict anus is Yoga way, too
From:      Aare
Date:       1999/12/18
Newsgroups: depression
[More Headers]

On Sat, 18 Dec 1999 07:32:55 GMT, Lms wrote:
On 18 Dec 1999 06 :22:38 GMT, Hiroyuki Nishigaki wrote:

Dear, sir
some snipped stuff
I think you will begin to have peculiar happy lucky feeling
in a month or a few months little by little.
oh, I have a peculiar feeling, alright.
me, too.

Cden
smells a poser

Subject:    Re: To constrict anus is Yoga way, too
From:       Yzoe
Date:       1999/12/18
Message-ID:
Newsgroups: depression
[More Headers]

On 18 Dec 1999 06:22:38 GMT, Hiroyuki Nishigaki wrote:

Dear, sir

To constrict anus 100 times in succession and dent navel 100 times in PAHLEEZE!! Do you mind?

Subject:    Re: To constrict anus is Yoga way, too
From:       Aawa
Date:       1999/12/18
Message-ID:
Newsgroups: depression
[More Headers]

On 18 Dec 1999 06:22:38 GMT, Hiroyuki Nishigaki wrote:

Dear, sir

To constrict anus 100 times in succession and dent navel 100 times in succession after constricting anus is very simple. It is one of the secret ways of Yoga to strengthen body and heart, too. You do not need any implement. If you do so every-day, you will learn the trick soon. I think you will begin to have peculiar happy lucky feeling in a month or a few months little by little.

I have received the present today, too which one who has practiced it for a year sent to me. If you practice it, confirm the effect and teach it to someone, someone will owe much gratitude to you. If we can give joy to someone at first, some-one will give joy to us. I think it is a good medicine to prevent or cure depression.

Hiroyuki Nishigaki

I am ROFL just thinking about what kind of 'present' you get from constricting your anus 100 times!

Aawa

—Toto...I don't think we're in Kansas anymore.


Subject:    Re: To constrict anus is Yoga way, too
From:       Stez
Date:       Sat, 18 December 1999 10:33 AM EST
Message-ID:
Newsgroups: depression
[More Headers]

Oh!!
Thread has me laughing and crying. It has made my day.
Isn't it odd that the people in asd are the funniest bunch I know?
Stez, still wiping the tears.


Subject:    Re: To constrict anus is Yoga way, too
From:       Klud
Date:       Sat, 18 December 1999 11:51 AM EST
Message-ID:
Newsgroups: depression
[More Headers]

stop it!

you guys are killing me here!

it's not healthy to laugh so hard so eary in the morning. i'm working my way to getting my present.

Stez wrote in massage:

Oh!!

Thread has me laughing and crying. It has made my day.

Isn't it odd that the people in asd are the funniest bunch I know?

Stez, still wiping the tears.

Subject:    Re: To constrict anus is Yoga way, too
From:      Abea
Date:       1999/12/18 01:20 PM EST
Message-ID:
Newsgroups: depression
[More Headers]

Damn. I always seem to get everything backwards! For all these years, I've been constricting my navel, and denting my anus. No wonder I'm constipated and depressed!

Abea

Subject:    Re: To constrict anus is Yoga way, too
From:      Hiroyuki Nishigaki
Date:       1999/12/19 GMT
Message-ID:
Newsgroups: depression
[More Headers]

Hello Abea

To cure constipation is essential to cure depression. I will wrote about it in How to good-by depression 4-6. So, please, wait for a while. I had had the bad bowel movement, but I can go to stool a few times everyday now.

Subject:    Re: To constrict anus is Yoga way too
From:      Aawa
Date:      Sat, 18 December 1999 10:01 PM EST
Message-ID:
Newsgroups: depression

On 19 Dec 1999 02:30:51 GMT, Hiroyuki Nishigaki wrote:

Hello Abea

To cure constipation is essential to cure depression. I will wrote about it in How to good-by depression 4-6. So, please, wait for a while. I had had the bad bowel movement, but I can go to stool a few times everyday now.

What is this Crap?

Aawa

Toto I don't think we're in Kansas anymore

Subject:    Re: To constrict anus is Yoga way, too
From:      Abea
Date:      Sat, 18 December 1999 10:17 PM EST
Message-ID:
Newsgroups: depression

This is freakin' priceless!
ROFL!!!

Abea

Subject:    Re: To constrict anus is Yoga way, too
From:       Guy
Date:       Sat, 18 December 1999 11:29 PM EST
Message-ID:
Newsgroups: depression

x-no-archive: yes
posted only
Oh, God, my face hurts…I can't handle all these endorphins, please stop
Guy, really can't stop laughing
But I don't want to go among people?
remarked Aali.
Oh, you can't help that,? said the Bca,? we're all mad here. I'm mad. You're mad.?
How do you know I'm mad? said Aali.
You must be?, replied the Bca,? or you wouldn't have come here?

Subject:    Re: To constrict anus is Yoga way, too
From:       Hiroyuki Nishigaki
Date:       999/12/19
Message-ID:
Newsgroups: depression
[More Headers]

Dear Aare and Lms

The formal way to constrict anus and dent navel involves drinking a cup of water as soon as you get up and doing bowel movement 6 times everyday (every bowel movement is more than 5 minutes. No excrement is Ok. Twice in the morning, twice in the daytime, twice in the evening). If you are interested in, you had better do so, too.

It is effective to strengthen body and heart that you only constrict anus 100 times If you are busy.

Dear, sir

some snipped stuff

I think you will begin to have peculiar happy lucky feeling in a month or a few months little by little.

Oh, I have a peculiar feeling, alright.

Hiroyuki Nishigaki
Spirit bless you!


Subject:    Re: To constrict anus is Yoga way too
From:      Xyuk
Date:      Sat, 18 December 1999 01:54 PM EST
Message-ID:
Newsgroups: depression

Hiroyuki Nishigaki wrote:

You do not need any implement.

Ummmmm.... I really hadn't anticipated using any implements

Subject:    Re: To constrict anus is Yoga way, too
From:       Lmt
Date:       Sun, 19 December 1999 10:51 PM EST
Message-ID:
Newsgroups: depression

On 18 Dec 1999 06:22:38 GMT, Hiroyuki Nishigaki wrote:

Dear, sir

To constrict anus 100 times in succession and dent navel 100 times in succession after constricting anus is very simple. It is one of the secret ways of Yoga to strengthen body and heart, too. You do not need any implement. If

And ladies, don't forget to do your Kegel exercise!

Lmt

I'd rather regret what I have done than wish for that which I didn't.-Me


Subject:    Re: To constrict anus is Yoga way, too
From:       Vwt
Date:       Sun, 19 December 1999 11:12 PM EST
Message-ID:

"Lmt" wrote:

And ladies, don't forget to do your Kegel exercises! ;)

The only time I think to do those is while sitting in church. Is that wrong?

—Vwt

"There's no insult like the truth."-Charlie Peacock

Subject:    Re: To constrict anus is Yoga way, too
From:       Lmt
Date:       Sun, 19 December 1999 11:50 PM EST
Message-ID:

On Sun, 19 Dec 1999 23:12:08-0500, Vwoh wrote:

> "Lmt" wrote:
> And ladies, don't forget to do your Kegel exercises! ;)
> The only time I think to do those is while sitting in
> church. Is that wrong?
> Yes. You are going strait to hell. ;)
> I do them at red lights and while I read email.

Lmt

I'd rather regret what I have done than wish for that
which I didn't.-Me

Subject:    Re: To constrict anus is Yoga way, too
From:       Rsuz
Date:       1999/12/20
Message-ID:
Newsgroups: depression
[More Headers]

This stuff is great for depressed people. I couldn't stop
laughing!

Damn it I nearly considered it-anything to get rid of the
damn depression!

But seriously having funny people like this around is good
for us!

I've heard laughing is good therapy

"Lmt" wrote:

On 18 Dec 1999 06:22:38 GMT, Hiroyuki Nishigaki wrote:
Dear, sir

To constrict anus 100 times in succession and dent navel 100 times in succession after constricting anus is very simple. It is one of the secret ways of Yoga to strengthen body and heart, too. You do not need any implement. If

And ladies, don't forget to do your Kegel exercises! ;)

Lmt
Ghis

I'd rather regret what I have done than wish for that which I didn't.-Me

Subject:   Re: To constrict anus is Yoga way, too
From:      Rsh
Date:      1999/12/20
Message-ID:
Newsgroups: depression
[More Headers]

And ladies, don't forget to do your Kegel exercises! ;)

The only time I think to do those is while sitting in church. Is that wrong?

The only time I think to do it is when I see the words "constrict your anus."

Shi

Subject:    Re: To constrict anus is Yoga way, too
From:       Lmt
Date:       1999/12/20
Message-ID:
Newsgroups: depression
[More Headers]

On 18 Dec 1999 06:22:38 GMT, Hiroyuki Nishigaki wrote:

Dear, sir

To constrict anus 100 times in succession and dent navel 100 times in succession after constricting anus is very simple. It is one of the secret ways of Yoga to strengthen body and heart, too. You do not need any implement. If

And ladies, don't forget to do your Kegel exercises! ;)

Lmt

I'd rather regret what I have done than wish for that which I didn't.-Me

Subject:    Re: To constrict anus is Yoga way, too
From:       Hiroyuki Nishigaki
Date:       1999/12/20
Message-ID:
Newsgroups: depression
[More Headers]

Hello Cdis

I sent my reply to you by E-mail, but it could not reach you. Unknown, Could not deliver. How are you getting along?

I am sorry that I wonder if you have committed suicide. My reply to you has been opened here and seem to have made many people laugh. Please?contribute here if you have no problem.

Subject:    Re: How to good-by depression 2
From:      Cdis
Date:      1999/12/16
Message-ID:
Newsgroups: depression
[More Headers]

Hiroyuki Nishigaki wrote in message news:

Hello

I have also constricted my anus and dented my navel 100 times in succession almost everyday for about 18 years after I was taught by him. As a result, I have grown 10-20 years younger. Furthermore, I can overcome the stress of various complains which are the causes of depression. I owe much gratitude to him now.

How old were you, and how old are you now?

I'm intrigued...just how do you constrict the anus? Is it like trying to hold it in when you desperately need to do a poo? Or does it involve the use of some kind of anal bull-worker or dumbells?

Hiroyuki Nishigaki
Spirit bless you!

Subject:    Re: To constrict anus is Yoga way, too
From:       Cdis
Date:       1999/12/20
Message-ID:
Newsgroups: depression
[More Headers]

Hi Hiroyuki

I am still here…alive and well and still wondering about this whole anal constriction mullarky.

You have to realise that anal exercises are an amusing (or erotic) concept for most of us in the west.

I'm sure that our laughter wasn't intended to offend…please just put it down to our warped sense of humour.

I hope you and your sphincter remain healthy.

Cdis

Hiroyuki Nishigaki wrote in message news:.

Hello Cdis

I sent my reply to you by E-mail, but it could not reach you. Unknown, Could not deliver How are you getting along?

I am sorry that I wonder if you have committed suicide. My reply to you have been opened here and seem to have made many people laugh. Please?contribute here if you have no problem.

Subject:   Re: How to good-by depression 2
From:      Cdis
Date:          1999/12/16
Message-ID:
Newsgroups: depression
[More Headers]

Hiroyuki Nishigaki wrote in message news:

Hello

I have also constricted my anus and dented my navel 100 times in succession almost everyday for about 18 years after I was taught by him. As a result,I have grown 10-20 years younger. Furthermore, I can overcome the stress of various complains which are the causes of depression. I owe much gratitude to him now.

How old were you, and how old are you now?

I'm intrigued…just how do you constrict the anus? Is it like trying to hold it in when you desperately need to do a poo? Or does it involve the use of some kind of anal bull-worker or dumbells?

Hiroyuki Nishigaki
Spirit bless you!


Subject:   Re: To constrict anus is Yoga way, too
From:      Vwom
Date:      Mon, 20 December 1999 03:11 PM EST
Message-ID:
Newsgroups: depression

On 20 Dec 1999 12:55:51 GMT, Hiroyuki Nishigaki said:

My reply to you have been opened here and seem to have made many people laugh. Please?

Hiroyuki, you are making a classic error: not understanding your audience.

You posted here with very little introduction, presenting a concept that is incredibly far outside of our usual thinking.

I suspect that you did not read the posts in this newsgroup long enough to understand what our culture here is. That's an important thing to do.


Subject:    How to good-by depression 3
From:       Hiroyuki Nishigaki
Date:       1999/12/21
Message-ID:
Newsgroups: depression
[More Headers]

Hello

I think the cause of depression or cancer is the stress of the complain?

about opposite sex (for example, divorce, big lost love), son or daughter, parents, boss, money, work or post.

If we had such a complain, we have bad complexion, bad bowel movement, bad sleeping, bad appetite, bad sex, stiff shoulder, strange feeling of finger or subtle lamp where cancer will happen in 3-5 years.

As a result, we may go to doctors. But, in most cases, no problem in medical respect at first.3-5 years later we will go to doctors. Then cancer will happen completely. Or, we may be suffering from depression. We will become cynical, lose a temper or withdraw ourselves

So, I think we had better make efforts to have good complexion and live with joy, pleasure, gratitude if we want not to be suffering from cancer or depression or want to cure it.

I think firm and soft strong abdomen, waist, buttocks, inside and outside of thigh, legs can generate much good energy(for example, the energy to make ourselves laugh heartily) to have good complexion and live with joy, pleasure, gratitude and to resist the stress of the complaint. Dear KLS contributed to How to good-by depression 2 "thank you! I needed to laugh, and you just cracked me up!". Dear Kls is happy because dear Kls has had fairly firm and soft strong abdomen, waist, buttocks, inside and outside of thigh, legs so that dear Kls can have laughed heartily at last. Dear Kls has not get stuck completely. I will write about how to clean up the pipe in our bodies where the energy of laugh flows later. But. we have to generate and multiply the energy of laugh at first.

If we had flabby or poor weak abdomen, waist, buttocks, inside and outside of thigh, legs, we will lack in our energy to have good complexion and live with joy, pleasure, gratitude so that we can not resist the stress of the complaint. Then, we are apt to have bad complexion, bad bowel movement, bad sleeping, bad appetite, bad sex, stiff shoulder, strange feeling of finger or subtle lamp. We will become cynical, lose a temper or withdraw into ourselves. We begin to throw much damn to ourselves and others. As a result, we will end up receiving much more damn from ourselves and others.

We are apt to go anywhere by car and eat too much now. In most cases, we are apt not to strengthen abdomen, waist, buttocks, inside and outside of thigh, legs so that we are apt to have flabby or poor weak abdomen, waist, buttocks, inside and outside of thigh, legs. Then, we have little good energy to resist the stress of the complaint and will be beaten by cancer or depression easily.

To constrict anus 100 times in succession and dent navel 100 times in succession after constricting anus everyday is only one example for us to strengthen waist, buttocks, inside and outside of thigh, legs so that we can have good complexion, live with joy, pleasure, gratitude and can resist the stress of the complaint. I think simple Tibetan exercises which are described in the book with the title-Ancient Secret of The Fountain of Youth (by Harbor Press?Inc) are effective to prevent or cure depression little by little, too because these exercises stimulate and strengthen flabby or poor abdomen, waist, buttocks, inside and outside of thigh, legs. In addition, we can breathe deeply naturally.

Hiroyuki Nishigaki<br>
Spirit bless you!

Subject:    How to good-by depression 4
From:      Hiroyuki Nishigaki
Date:       1999/12/22
Message-ID:
Newsgroups: depression
[More Headers]

Hello Xyuk

Have you still made fun of me or a little serious question? I have not such a video or half-hour info-mercial.

But, owing to your question, I have thought of one idea. Some people and I will gather and make such a video a year later if some people try to constrict anus 100 times and dent navel 100 times everyday (in addition, drink a cup of water as soon as get up and do bowel movement six times everyday), begin to be able to have peculiar happy lucky, good complexion, good bowel movement, good appetite, good sex, good sleeping, soft shoulder little by little in a month or a few months, begin to confirm the effect and can graduate from The University of Depression a year later without failing the test(which may result in a misery such as suicide, cancer or entering the mental hospital).

Furthermore, Some people and I will found a club such as Anus 100 Club if possible. Then, we will make such a video in which all of us perform and talk about own overcoming depression. We will give such a video for free to someone who is suffering from big anxiety and depression. We may be on the air.

I think God deals with us fairly. We can not have only good luck and can not have only misfortune. Good luck and misfortune are apt to happen to us every 3-5years (at most 10 years) in turn. Those who have begun to be proud and look down upon other people are apt to ruin in 3-5years (at most 10 years).

When we fall into misfortune, we had better not to ran away from it desperately. If we accept it calmly, it will ran away from us in 3-5years (at most 10 years). That is to say, we will drown in the water when we flounder desperately under water. When we fall into deep water, we can come to the surface naturally and escape if we sink into obediently.

For 3-5years (at most 10 years), we had better make friends with our misfortune which is the cause of depression, cancer, suicide. Then, we had better find and enjoy different joys and pleasures outside the misfortune practicing some exercise to strengthen our bodies and hearts. While living so for 3-5years (at most 10 years), misfortune will ran away from us and those who have tortured us will ruin by cancer, insanity or some big failure and so on. Your comeback will be the biggest revenge if you want to revenge those who have tortured you. They will not be able to look at your face. f you ruin by yourself now, those who have tortured you can have accomplished their purposes. So, we had better begin to stand up for ourselves.

The 70 year old man who taught me constricting anus and denting navel 18 years ago have lived under the difficult circumstance for long years. I think he would die of cancer or be suffering from depression if he did not constrict anus and dent navel. He often says to me "Now, I can say that I am happy and have a good luck after all. All of those who had looked down upon me have ruined already".

Hello Ab.

We had better constrict anus and dent navel at ease. We can do so in a boring meeting, subway or at red lights like dear Lmt. Furthermore, We are apt to waist time to indulge in self-pity, depression or hate. We are apt to always throw much damn to ourselves and others and end up receiving much more damn from ourselves and others. We can cut away a little of such a time, and constrict anus and dent navel. The day when you are busy, you had better only constrict anus 20 times at least. Or, you had better constrict anus 100 times and dent navel 100 times for 2 days. If you do nothing for 3 days, it will begin to make your peculiar happy lucky ran away from you and begin to make you indulge in self-pity, depression, and hate. So, you had better practice a little of so-called strange exercise at least every 2 days.

Subject:    Re: How to good-by depression
From:       Xyuk
Date:       1999/12/21
Message-ID:
Newsgroups: depression
[More Headers]

Is there an anal constriction video and half-hour info-mercial?


Subject:    Re: How to good-by depression
From:       Xyuko
Date:       1999/12/13
Message-ID:
Newsgroups: depression
[More Headers]

Ab wrote:

I once dented my anus in the Navy. I was put on constrictive duty.

This happened 100 times. Bahahaha!

I though your anus was a planet....

Hiroyuki Nishigaki
Spirit bless you!


Subject:    Re: How to good-by depression 4
From:       Cdis
Date:       1999/12/22
Message-ID:
Newsgroups: depression
[More Headers]

snigger snigger

Subject:    Re: How to good-by depression 4
From:       Cdis
Date:       1999/12/22
Message-ID:
Newsgroups: depression
[More Headers]

Hi Hiroyuki

I am so sorry you feel like we are mocking you. You need to understand that the anus is a kind of tabboo subject for many of us in our societies and cultures (not for everybody, but for many).

Some of us deal with this kind of thing by humor. I mean it *IS* funny. It is such a shame you can't appreciate how funny it is. The comic delivery couldn't be better.

You have helped me by making me smile (and nearly wet myself once). I really don't mean that to disrespect you, because you have had a positive effect on my life by this post.

Thanks

Cdis


Subject:    Re: How to good-by depression 4
From:       Mnd
Date:       Wed, 22 December 1999 03:24 PM EST
Message-ID:
Newsgroups: depression
[More Headers]

In article, Hiroyuki Nishigaki wrote:

Furthermore, Some people and I will found a club such as Anus100 Club

Let me know if you do, I'll give you a plug.

Mnd


Subject:     Re: How to good-by depression 4
From:        Lmel
Date:        1999/12/22
Message-ID:
Newsgroups: depression
[More Headers]

I hereby nominate RM as president of the Anus 100 Club.

On 22 Dec 1999 18:46:17 GMT, Hiroyuki Nishigaki wrote:

Furthermore, some people and I will found a club such as Anus 100 Club if possible. Then, we will make such a video in which all of us perform and talk about own overcoming depression. We will give such a video for free to someone who is suffering from big anxiety and depression. We may be on the air.

—Lmel

It may be that your sole purpose in life is simply to serve as a warning to others.


Subject:     Re: How to good-by depression 4
From:        Rsta
Date:        1999/12/22
Message-ID:
Newsgroups: depression
[More Headers]

Hiroyuki Nishigaki wrote:

clipped a little

if some people try to constrict anus 100 times and dent navel 100 times everyday (in addition, drink a cup of water as soon as get up and do bowel movement six times everyday), begin to be able to have peculiar happy lucky, good complexion, good bowel movement, good appetite, good sex, good sleeping, soft shoulder little by little in a month or a few months, begin to confirm the effect and can graduate from The University of Depression a year later without failing the test(which may result in a misery such as suicide, cancer or entering the mental hospital)

It would save a lot of time if one could constrict the anus and dent the navel at the same time (100 times). Is this acceptable?

clipped the rest

Subject:    Re: How to good-by depression 4
From:       Aawa
Date:       1999/12/22
Message-ID:
Newsgroups: depression
[More Headers]

On 22 Dec 1999 18:46:17 GMT, Hiroyuki Nishigaki Furthermore, Some people and I will found a club such as Anus 100 Club if possible. Then, we will make such a video in which all of us perform and talk about own overcoming depression. We will give such a video for free to someone who is suffering from big anxiety and depression. We may be on the air.

I can suggest a few charter members for that Anus club...

Aawa

—Toto...I don't think we're in Kansas anymore.


Subject:    Re: How to good-by depression 4
From:       Abok
Date:       1999/12/22
Message-ID:
Newsgroups: depression
[More Headers]

Hiroyuki Nishigaki wrote:

Furthermore, Some people and I will found a club such as Anus 100 Club if possible. Then, we will make such a video in which all of us perform and talk about own overcoming depression. We will give such a video for free to someone who is suffering from big anxiety and depression. We may be on the air.

Somehow, I don't think I want to be downwind of that program when it does air.

Ijam

—"Once you become aware of this force for unity in life, you can't ever forget it. It becomes part of everything you do."
—John Bcol 'Meditations'
Visit The Abok Cafe

Subject:    Re: How to good-by depression 4
From:        Mnd
Date:        Wed, 22 December 1999 05:30 PM EST
Message-ID:
Newsgroups: depression
[More Headers]

> I mean, what if the video really stinks?
> Anus 100 Club my ass!


Subject:    Re: How to good-by depression 4
From:        Aare
Date:        Wed, 22 December 1999 06:43 PM EST
Message-ID:
Newsgroups: depression
[More Headers]

On Wed, 22 December 1999 17:30:33-0500, Mnd wrote:

> I mean, what if the video really stinks?
> Anus 100 Club my ass!
> if you haven't figured it out yet, you're being trolled.

Cden

i may not be the sharpest pencil in the box,
but at least i have a point. Cden knapp

Subject:    Re: How to good-by depression 4
From:       Hiroyuki Nishigaki
Date:       1999/12/23
Message-ID:
Newsgroups:
[More Headers]

Hello Cdis

As you advise me, that is a delicate subject. I think I have to write about it with humor and delicacy even though it is one of the secret Yoga ways. It is not only one subject which I will write about. It is one of the subjects which I will write about.

I never think you are mocking me. Whenever I remember 96 contributions, I always begin to smile and laugh.

Especially on Dec 22,I laughed and nearly wetted myself, too remembering your contribution "You have helped me by making me smile (and nearly wet myself once)".You have made me nearly wet. too. I imagine you have had some **?I have had some **,too?

Merry Christmas and Happy New Year

Sincerely. Hiroyuki Nishigaki

Subject:    Re: How to good-by depression 4
From:       Cdis
Date:       Wed, 22 December 1999 03:32 PM EST
Message-id:

Hi Hiroyuki

I am so sorry you feel like we are mocking you. You need to understand that the anus is a kind of tabboo subject for many of us in our societies and cultures (not for everybody, but for many).

Some of us deal with this kind of thing by humor. I mean it *IS* funny. It is such a shame you can't appreciate how funny it is. The comic delivery couldn't be better.

You have helped me by making me smile (and nearly wet myself once). I really don't mean that to disrespect you, because you have had a positive effect on my life by this post.

Thanks Cdis

Hiroyuki Nishigaki
Spirit bless you!

Subject:    Re: How to good-by depression 4
From:       Ijtf
Date:       1999/12/23
Message-ID:
Newsgroups: depression
[More Headers]

Mnd wrote in article

In article Hiroyuki Nishigaki wrote:

Furthermore, Some people and I will found a club such as Anus 100 Club Will membership be constricted?

Abri

Subject:  Re: How to good-by depression 4
From:     Dfg
Date:     1999/12/23
Message-ID:
Newsgroups: depression
[More Headers]

Ijtf wrote:

> Mnd wrote in article
> In article, Hiroyuki Nishigaki wrote:
> Furthermore, Some people and I will found a club such as
> Anus 100 Club Will membership be constricted?
>
> Abri

In that clubroom I'd worry about astutes.


Subject:  Re: How to good-by depression 4
From:     Rst
Date:     1999/12/23
Message-ID:
Newsgroups: depression
[More Headers]

Abok wrote:

> Hiroyuki Nishigaki wrote:
> Furthermore, Some people and I will found a club such as
> Anus 100 Club if possible. Then, we will make such a video
> in which all of us perform and talk about own overcoming
> depression. We will give such a video for free to someone who
> is suffering from big anxiety and depression. We may be on
> the air.

Somehow, I don't think I want to be downwind of that program when it does air.

Dial 1-800-ANUS-100 and make your pledge now.

Rst

Subject:    Re: How to good-by depression 4
From:       Cdis
Date:       1999/12/24
Message-ID:
Newsgroups: depression
[More Headers]

Ijtf wrote in article:

Mnd wrote in article
Hiroyuki Nishigaki wrote:
Furthermore, Some people and I will found a club such as Anus 100 Club Will membership be constricted?
Would I have to grease any palms in order to get in? Sounds interesting…I might have to probe a bit further.

Subject:    Re: How to good-by depression 4
From:       Hiroyuki Nishigaki
Date:       1999/12/24
Message-ID:
Newsgroups: depression
[More Headers]

Hello Dfre, Aare
Let's strain our small brains about the following problems, too one after another while beating our brains out not to be

constricted by the causes of depression or cancer one after another. Two heads are better than one. I think the following problems will keep on being our funny, pleasant assignments for us until next year Christmas.

To gather and meet us a year later with fun and laugh if possible, we have to emancipate from the present constriction by then. Don't let's fail the test of The University of Depression.

Sincerely. Hiroyuki Nishigaki


From:      Dfgk
Date:      Thu, 23 December 1999 03:01 PM EST
Message-id:

Ijtf wrote:

Mnd wrote in article,

Hiroyuki Nishigaki wrote:

Furthermore, Some people and I will found a club such as Anus 100 Club Will membership be constricted?

Abri

In that clubroom I'd worry about astutes.

Hiroyuki Nishigaki
Spirit bless you!

# Part 2 Turn to bay throwing away pride

Subject:    How to good-by depression 5
From:       Hiroyuki Nishigaki
Date:       1999/12/27
Message-ID:
Newsgroups: depression
[More Headers]

Hello

**Some leading disciple of Buddha had never complained about his poor living and meditated earnestly.**

Some leading disciple of Buddha never complained about whatever foods he was given by ordinary other people or however rudely he was given foods by ordinary other people 2500 years ago in India. He approached ordinary other people calmly and modestly as if he had been clear Moon. He never complained about whatever clothes he wore, too. He enjoyed wearing clothes that were made of thrown-away rag. When a Hunsen's patient gave him food, a rotten finger of a Hunsen's patient dropped into his bowl together with food, he ate both the food and the rotten finger in his bowl calmly.

Buddha told him "You do not have to walk around other ordinary people's houses to gather foods because you become old. You had better sit beside me and eat foods with me everyday which my followers bring to me. You had better wear neat clothes which my followers bring to me, too".

Buddha asked him why he did so. Then, he replied "Someone will be able to become selfless and calm down at night if someone of future generation knows that such a leading disciple of Buddha as me kept on gathering and eating poor meals, wearing poor clothes, and meditating in the wood seriously everyday in spite of old age. In this respect, I have kept on doing an act of charity for many people of future generation. I have been giving good feeling(power) to many people of future generation". Buddha was very pleased to hear his answer.

### The priest of Jaina religion in India lives with his body daubed by mud.

The priests of Jaina (spelling?) religion in India daub mud on all over their bodies and live in such a way. Jaina religion was founded 2500 years ago in India. It has 400-500 thousand rich followers like merchants of jewelry. I saw they were daubing mud on all over their bodies in front of some stream when I visited India 20 years ago. At first, I thought they were washing with mud of some stream. But, I mistook the meaning of such a way because they were walking in a town with their bodies daubed by mud. To practice becoming selfless, abandoning themselves and calming down (being patient) under difficult conditions, they seem to be living in such a way. Such a way seems like writing "STUPID" with paint on forehead and walking calmly in a town.

Most of us or all of us will be driven to the last ditch or humiliate ourselves at least once or twice in the course of life. If we always get upset, indulge in self-pity(or depression or hate), break down into tears, or go out of the way in such a case, we will ruin. While we are letting it take the course of nature for a while and calm down under difficult conditions, body-response will happen to you. Then, you will tempt the fate at your perils following your body-response to your surroundings. I often wish I could live writing "STUPID" with paint on my forehead in Japan. Some day, I will visit India again and walk with my body daubed by mud.

Subject:   How to good-by depression 5
From:       Hiroyuki Nishigaki
Date:        1999/12/25
Message-ID:
Newsgroups: depression
[More Headers]

Hello

**Sink in the hell willingly and you can break through the bottom of the hell. Welcome an insult to you sometimes a month**

According to the Buddhist precepts, followers had better (1)eat once by noon (2)not eat animal food or animal-protein (3)not drink alcohol, not smoke (4)not make love with opposite sex (5)not kill (6)not thieve (7)not tell a lie (8)not make up (9)sleep on the mat on the earth(not sleep or sit on gorgeous bed or chair)-on 8th, 14th, 15th, 23rd, 29th and 30th day every month as possible.

In a broad sense, (8)and (9) mean being well content with our present lives, being modest, compromise, not glossing ourselves or not being competitive. For example, I sometimes behave as the foot of some meeting, of some party, or of some group when I attend it. I behave as if I were a blockhead or ill, too. I welcome an insult to me or a contempt for me. I am pleased to be beaten on such a day. I sometimes follow these precepts as possible. Then, I feel better and relieved. You had better try only for a day. You will surely feel so, too. You will think reading my contribution pays you well.

That is to say, we don't have to bear a heavy load of competition, of ranking, of love, of trouble, of disease, of complaint, of grudge, of fear, of irritation, of self-pity, of guilt and of much sadness everyday. Sometimes, we had better throw away such a heavy load. How to throw away it is not to run away from it but to welcome it.

When we fall into deep water, we will die if we flounder desperately to save under water. If we sink in deep water obediently, we will come to the surface automatically. Sometimes, we had better welcome so-called hell and sink in it as deeply as possible. Then, ironically, we can break through the bottom of the hell or the hell will run away from us. Such a way is to make friends with danger or death, too. A hero, general, founder, pioneer and enterpriser are good at such a way. One of the famous general of old age said "if we strive to save, we will be killed. If we strive to die, we will be saved".

I think we can sometimes cure a terminal cancer or a depression if we don't follow the advice of doctor. My another acquaintance ran works and cured a terminal cancer of spinal cord. His doctor said that he would die in a month.

He said to me about 3 years ago "I decided not to die on the bed of hospital but to die working in my works. I threw away medicine". He left the hospital and began to work in his works. He could walk only 50 mm at first. He could cured the incurable cancer of spinal cord but some small holes had remained on his spinal cord and his spinal cord had became bent.

Subject:    Re: How to good-by depression
From:      Abok
Date:      1999/12/13
Message-ID: [More Headers]
Newsgroups: depression

I think it is effective to constrict your anus 100 times in succession
Welllllllllllllll...first you'd need to remove your head from there.

Ijam

Say it out loud. I'm depressed and I'm proud. well....just depressed
OWWWW!!!!!! I don't feel good...
In a funk but always funky, and with plenty of soul.

Hiroyuki Nishigaki
Spirit bless you!

Subject:    Re: How to good-by depression 5
From:      Ijen
Date:      1999/12/25
Message-ID:
Newsgroups: depression

Hiroyuki Nishigaki wrote:

[snip]

Are you using some sort of auto-translator? It's coming across kind of weird.

not make love with opposite sex

So does that mean homosexual sex is ok?


Subject:    Re: How to good-by depression 5
From:       Lmu
Date:       1999/12/25
Message-ID:
Newsgroups: depression
[More Headers]

Ijen wrote:

Hiroyuki Nishigaki wrote:
[snip]
not make love with opposite sex
So does that mean homosexual sex is ok?
you know.... I was wondering the same thing...


Subject:    Re: How to good-by depression 5
From:       Rstu
Date:       1999/12/25
Message-ID:
Newsgroups: depression
[More Headers]

Ijen wrote:

Hiroyuki Nishigaki wrote:
[snip]
Are you using some sort of auto-translator? It's coming across kind of weird.

not make love with opposite sex

So does that mean homosexual sex is ok?

When properly done, yes.

Auto-translators, however, really remove much of the meaning.

Rstu


Subject:    Re: How to good-by depression 5
From:       Abt
Date:       1999/12/26
Message-ID:
Newsgroups: depression
[More Headers]

On 25 Dec 1999 16:08:20 GMT, Hiroyuki Nishigaki wrote:

According to the Buddhist precepts, followers had better?

Those are the rules for monks and nuns.

Are you thinking of joining a monastery?

—Abev.


Subject:    Re: How to good-by depression 5
From:       Hiroyuki Nishigaki
Date:       1999/12/27
Message-ID:
Newsgroups: depression
[More Headers]

Hello

Such Buddhist precepts were followed by the followers in India 2500 years ago. Those were only basic rules for monks and nuns. There were 200-300 rules for monks and nuns. I am not thinking of joining a monastery.

Hiroyuki Nishigaki
Spirit bless you!


Subject:    Re: How to good-by depression 5
From:       Abt
Date:       1999/12/27
Message-ID:
Newsgroups: depression
[More Headers]

On 27 Dec 1999 19:03:27 GMT, Hiroyuki Nishigaki wrote:

I am not thinking of joining a monastery.

Then follow householder or bodhisattva rules. In Buddhism, proper practice is important. Study more dharma. You are making karma.


Subject:    How to good-by depression 6
From:       Hiroyuki Nishigaki
Date:       1999/12/27
Message-ID:
Newsgroups: depression
[More Headers]

Hello

**Some leading disciple of Buddha had never complained about his poor living and meditated earnestly**

Some leading disciple of Buddha never complained about whatever foods he was given by ordinary other people or however rudely he was given foods by ordinary other people 2500 years ago in India. He approached ordinary other people calmly and modestly as if he had been clear Moon. He never complained about whatever clothes he wore, too. He enjoyed wearing clothes which were made of thrown-away rag. When a Hunsen's patient gave him food, a rotten finger of a Hunsen's patient dropped into his bowl together with food, he ate both the food and the rotten finger in his bowl calmly.

Buddha told him "You do not have to walk around other ordinary people's houses to gather foods because you become old. You had better sit beside me and eat foods with me everyday which my followers bring to me. You had better wear neat clothes that my followers bring to me, too".

Buddha asked him why he did so. Then, he replied "Someone will be able to become selfless and calm down at night if someone of future generation knows that such a leading disciple of Buddha as me kept on gathering and eating poor meals, wearing poor clothes, and meditating in the wood seriously everyday in spite of old age. In this respect, I have kept on doing an act of charity for many people of future generation. I have been giving good feeling (power) to many people of future generation". Buddha was very pleased to hear his answer.

### The priest of Jaina religion in India lives with his body daubed by mud

The priests of Jaina(spelling?) religion in India daub mud on all over their bodies and live in such a way. Jaina religion was founded 2500 years ago in India. It has 400-500 thousand rich followers like merchants of jewelry.

I saw they were daubing mud on all over their bodies in front of some stream when I visited India 20 years ago. At first, I thought they were washing with mud of some stream. But, I mistook the meaning of such a way because they were walking in a town with their bodies daubed by mud. To practice becoming selfless, abandoning themselves and calming down (being patient) under difficult conditions, they seem to be living in such a way. Such a way seems like writing "STUPID" with paint on forehead and walking calmly in a town.

Most of us or all of us will be driven to the last ditch or humiliate ourselves at least once or twice in the course of life. If we always get upset, indulge in self-pity(or depression or hate), break down into tears, or go out of the way in such a case, we will ruin. While we are letting it take the course of nature for a while and calm down under difficult conditions, body-response will happen to you. Then, you will tempt the fate at your perils following your body-response to your surroundings. I often wish I could live writing "STUPID" with paint on my forehead. Some day, I will visit India again and walk with my body daubed by mud.

Hello Ijen, Lmud, Tstu and Cdoc

Thank you for your kind advices. Not to make love with opposite sex does

not mean homosexual is OK.

My auto-translator versioned up to TOFEL 597 about 5 years ago. But, it is the used auto-translator. The above mentioned English sentence is the limits of its abilities. Excuse for its poor abilities. So, please, understand some strange line of each How to good-by depression remembering all of How to good-by depression 1-if possible. I have tried to understand some difficult line of your contribution correctly as possible remembering all your about 100 contributions, too.

In this respect, I say thank you to dear Cdis. Dear Cdis wrote "You have helped me by making me smile (and nearly wet myself once). I really don't mean that to disrespect you, because you have had a positive effect on my life by this post". t is because Dear Cdis read my poor English contributions and nearly wetted once. Thank you.

Hiroyuki Nishigaki
Spirit bless you!

Subject:    How to good-by depression 7
From:       Hiroyuki Nishigaki
Date:       1999/12/29
Message-ID:
Newsgroups: depression
[More Headers]

Hello

**A petty tyrant**

Mr.Carlos Castaneda wrote 12 best-seller books about the ancient Inca secret knowledge that was taught by his teacher, don Juan Matus. His teacher, don Juan Matus said in the book with the title-The Fire From Within by Mr.Carlos Castaneda "A petty tyrant is a tormentor. Someone who either holds the power of life and death over warriors or simply annoys them to distraction".

"The new seers saw fit to head their classification with the primal source of energy, the one and only ruler in the universe, and they called it simply the tyrant(The Eagles, the black spirit, the black energy of the universe). The most fearsome, tyrannical men are buffoons (involving other color energies of the universe, the other color spirits and ally); consequently, they were classified as a petty tyrant. There were two sub-classes of minor petty tyrant. The first subclass consisted of the petty tyrants who persecute and inflict misery but without actually causing anybody's death. They were called little petty tyrant. The second consisted of the petty tyrant who are only exasperating and bothersome to no end. They were called small-fry petty tyrant, or teensy-weeny petty tyrants"(The Fire From Within).

I think that complaint (about opposite sex-divorce-big lost love-discord, son or daughter, health, parents, money, work or post), devils, dirty energy body of other, our dirty energy(stickiness, the fever of depression, coldness, numb-ness), eating too much, and bad complexion are petty tyrants (buffoons) or little petty tyrant or small-fry petty tyrant, too.

Furthermore, I think unhappy-unhealthy-inefficient people and founders, big men, pioneers, enterprisers who will become disgraced in 3-5 years seem to become a little petty tyrant or small-fry petty tyrant because they are apt to perse-cute or anger or bother other people to no end. They are not grateful but a grumbler. They are proud or careless. They take so many liberties.

A petty tyrant, little petty tyrant, small-fry petty tyrant have bad complexion, bad bowel movement, bad appetite, bad sleeping, bad sex, stiff shoulder, poor or flabby abdomen and rough breath. They seem as if they made very effort to transmit their pains to other people. They seem as if they were epidemic germs.

Don Juan Matus said to Mr.Carlos Castaneda "To be defeated by a small-fry petty tyrant is not deadly, but devastating. The degree of mortality, in a figurative sense, is almost as high. By that I mean that warriors who succumb to a small-fry petty tyrant are obliterated by their own sense of failure and unworthiness. That spells high mortality to me. {How do you measure defeat? }. Anyone who joins the petty tyrant is defeated. To act in anger, without control and discipline, to have no forbearance, is to be defeated. {What happens after warriors are defeated? }. They either regroup themselves or they abandon the quest for knowledge (the third attention, silent knowledge, the spirit, moving assemblage point to the point of undoubt, shooting out the third attention from body, stopping breath automatically, arriving or looking at two different places at the same moment, voice without voice) and join the ranks of the petty tyrant for life"(The Fire From Within).

Hiroyuki Nishigaki
Spirit bless you!

Subject:   Re: How to good-by depression 7
From:      Aawa
Date:      1999/12/29
Message-ID:
Newsgroups: depression
[More Headers]

On Wed, 29 Dec 1999 03:31:35 GMT, Aare wrote:

> wow! what an improvement in your English!
> troll, troll, troll your bait...
> Oh, wait. i changed the words a little.
> Cden

Maybe he'll only get to 10, after that we're all toast anyway!

Aawa

—Toto…I don't think we're in Kansas anymore.


Subject:    Re: How to good-by depression 7
From:       Aare
Date:       Tue, 28 December 1999 10:31 PM EST
Message-ID:
Newsgroups:

> wow! what an improvement in your English!
> troll, troll, troll, your bait…
> Oh, wait. i change the words a little.
> Cden

On 29 Dec 1999 03:20:17 GMT, Hiroyuki Nishigaki wrote:

Hello
A petty tyrant
Mr.Carlos Castaneda wrote 12 best-seller books about the ancient Inca secret knowledge which was taught by his teacher, don Juan Matus. His teacher, don Juan Matus said in the book with the title-The Fire From Within by Mr.Carlos Castaneda "A petty tyrant is a tormentor.

Someone who either holds the power of life and death over warriors or simply annoys them to distraction".

"The new seers saw fit to head their classification with the primal source of energy, the one and only ruler in the universe, and they called it simply the tyrant(The Eagles, the black spirit, the black energy of the universe). The most fearsome, tyrannical men are buffoons (involving other color energies of the universe, the other color spirits and ally);

consequently, they were classified as a petty tyrant. There were two subclasses of minor petty tyrant. The first subclass consisted of the petty tyrants who persecute and inflict misery but without actually causing anybody's death. They were called little petty tyrant. The second consisted of the petty tyrant who are only exasperating and bothersome to no end. They were called small-fry petty tyrant, or teensy-weeny petty tyrants"(The Fire From Within).

I think that complaint (about opposite sex-divorce-big lost love-discord,

son or daughter, health, parents, money, work or post), devils, dirty energy body of other, our dirty energy(stickiness, the fever of depression, coldness, numbness), eating too much, and bad complexion are petty tyrants (buffoons) or little petty tyrant or small-fry petty tyrant, too.

Furthermore, I think unhappy-unhealthy-inefficient people and founders, big men, pioneers, enterprisers who will become disgraced in 3-5 years seem to become a little petty tyrant or small-fry petty tyrant because they are apt to persecute or anger or bother other people to no end. They are not grateful but a grumbler. They are proud or careless. They take so many liberties.

A petty tyrant, little petty tyrant, small-fry petty tyrant have bad complexion, bad bowel movement, bad appetite, bad sleeping, bad sex, stiff shoulder, poor or flabby abdomen and rough breath. They seem as if they made every effort to transmit their pains to other people. They seem as if they were epidemic germs.

Don Juan Matus said to Mr.Carlos Castaneda "To be defeated by a small-fry petty tyrant is not deadly, but devastating. The degree of mortality, in a figurative sense, is almost as high. By that I mean that warriors who succumb to a small-fry petty tyrant are obliterated by their own sense of failure and unworthiness. That spells high mortality to me. {How do you measure defeat? }. Anyone who joins the petty tyrant is defeated. To act in anger, without control and discipline, to have no forbearance, is to be defeated. {What happens after warriors are defeated? }. They either regroup themselves or they abandon the quest for knowledge(the third attention, silent knowledge, the spirit, moving assemblage point to the point of undoubt, shooting out the third attention from body, stopping breath automatically, arriving or looking at two different places at the same moment, voice without voice) and join the ranks of the petty tyrant for life"(The Fire From Within).

Hiroyuki Nishigaki
Spirit bless you!

Growing up is not something to hurry through.
I plan to spend the rest of my life on this project.Diane Wilson

Aare

Subject:          Re: How to good-by depression 7
From:     Hiroyuki Nishigaki
Date:        1999/12/29
Message-ID:
Newsgroups: depression
[More Headers]

Hi Aawa, Aare and other readers
You wrote; wow! What an improvement in your English. Thank you.

Please, teach me a quite strange line of my contribution from now on if possible.

Hiroyuki Nishigaki
Spirit bless you!

Subject:   Re: How to good-by depression 7
From:      Aawa
Date:       1999/12/29
Message-ID:
Newsgroups: depression
[More Headers]

Sacred medicine journeys, YEA!!!

Aawa-

Toto…I don't think we're in Kansas anymore.

Subject:   Re: How to good-by depression 7
From:      Hiroyuki Nishigaki
Date:       1999/12/30
Message-ID:
Newsgroups: depression
[More Headers]

Hi someone

Has someone of my readers tried to play the part of block-head or the unhappiest person only for a day? I think it has given peculiar happy lucky feeling to someone as well as constricting anus 100 times in succession and denting navel100 times in succession.

I behave all day as if I were a blockhead or the unhappiest person once a week or month. Welcome insults. I can feel relieved and relaxed.

Hiroyuki Nishigaki
Spirit bless you!

Subject:    How to good-by depression 8
From:       Hiroyuki Nishigaki
Date:       1999/12/30
Message-ID:
Newsgroups: depression
[More Headers]

Hello

While throwing away your self-importance temporarily and groveling before a petty tyrant, you make a strategy to win and wait for a good timing patiently for 3-5 years(or 10 years or a year).

According to the book-The Fire from Within by Mr.Carlos Castaneda, you had better welcome a petty tyrant when you meet a petty tyrant. To temper yourself and enjoy yourself, you had better take advantage of a petty tyrant.

While throwing away your self-importance temporarily, being pleased to be given a whipping by a petty tyrant and fulfilling a petty tyrant's most foolish demands, you had better watch a petty tyrant's weakness and make a well-thought strategy and wait for a good timing to win a petty tyrant patiently. According to the book-The Fire From Within, such a control, discipline, forbearance, timing are the attributes of warriorship.

Instead of indulging in self-pity or the wear and tear or hate, we had better begin to have such a brass nerve as we try to temper ourselves playing with a petty tyrant. Don't deal with a petty tyrant seriously. Play with a petty tyrant for 3-5 years (at most 10 years) or only for a year. In this respect, I think constricting anus 100 times in succession and denting navel 100 times in succession everyday can give us such a brass nerve as we try to temper ourselves playing with a petty tyrant. Playing the part of blockhead or the unhappiest person all day once a week or a month is a example of playing with a petty tyrant, too.

I think that complaint (about opposite sex-divorce-big lost love-discord, son or daughter, health, parents, money, work or post), devils, dirty energy body of other and our dirty energy(stickiness, the fever of depression, coldness, numbness) are petty tyrants (buffoons) or little petty tyrants or small-fry petty tyrants, too. Furthermore, I think unhappy-unhealthy-inefficient people and founders, big men, pioneers, enterprisers who will become disgraced in 3-5 years(or 10 years or a year) are apt to become little petty tyrants or small-fry petty tyrants because they are apt to persecute or anger or bother other people to no end. They are not grateful but a grumbler. They are proud or careless. They take so many liberties.

Fighting against a petty tyrant can give you the ability to meet and deal with the tyrant (Eagle, black energy, the strong black spirit) safely. Such a ability is bravery, patience, self-possession, humor, decision, loyalty and independence.

Happy lucky feeling is power. Mr.Carlos Castaneda's teacher, Don Juan Matus said in the book that the sum of happy lucky feeling can decide your destiny and how to live. You can shoot out your immaterial fiber or third attention to a petty tyrant from your abdomen only when you have happy lucky feeling. When you are given a whipping by a petty tyrant, you had better not lose the same happy lucky feeling as those of light spring breeze, abandon, largess, ruthless, clarity, sweetness, inner silence, kindness, humor, patience, rushing headlong as possible.

Under a difficult condition, we had better have the happy lucky feeling of our eyes, of our speaking and of our behaviors. In such a case, we can keep on burning the fire within our abdomens and can shoot out our immaterial fibers or third attention to a petty tyrant at a good timing to win a petty tyrant. If we are temporarily pleased to be given a whipping by a petty tyrant, we can end up neither making the fire within our bodies go out nor throwing away such a happy lucky feeling.

Hiroyuki Nishigaki
Spirit bless you!

Subject:    How to good-by depression 9
From:       Hiroyuki Nishigaki
Date:        1999/12/31
Message-ID:
Newsgroups: depression
[More Headers]

Happy New Year!

### Challenge to multiply happy lucky feeling under a difficult condition

But, when most of us meet a petty tyrant, most of us make the fire within abdomens go out, throw away such a happy lucky feeling, look older and indulge in self-pity, irritation, hate or undependable positive self-image. In such a case, bad complexion, bad bowel movement, bad appetite, bad sleeping, looking older, stiff shoulder, poor or flabby abdomen and rough breath happen to speaking and of behavior. In such a case, our immaterial fibers or third attention are confined to our bodies. We can not shoot out our immaterial fibers or third attention to a petty tyrant from our bodies so that we can neither judge a petty tyrant accurately nor win a petty tyrant.

If we are defeated by a petty tyrant, we will indulge in much more self-pity, irritation and hate. We will become cynical and withdraw into ourselves. Or, we will become a new petty tyrant or a new small-fry petty tyrant. Then, worse complexion, worse bowel movement, worse appetite, worse sleeping, worse sex, looking much older, stiffer shoulder, and rougher breath happen to us. As a result, we will not be able to shoot out our immaterial fibers or third attention so that we will become unhappy-unhealthy-inefficient like a teethless tiger. Then, we may be suffering from depression so that we may enter mental hospital, commit suicide or be suffering from cancer, heart disease or paralysis sooner or later. A petty tyrant will accomplish his purpose to defeat us completely at last.

If you want to become a happy-healthy-efficient man, a warrior or a man of knowledge, you have to multiply the happy lucky feeling or mood (power) about your thought, eyes, voice, behavior in spite of your living in the difficult ordinary world for the purpose of being able to shoot out your immaterial fiber or third attention to an object. If you throw away such a happy lucky feeling and can not multiply such a happy lucky feeling under a difficult condition, such a happy lucky feeling is not yours but a borrowed thing.

I think "Those who can multiply happy lucky feeling under a difficult condition have a qualification of powerful man, of wisc man, of a patient man.

It is a statesman that can make many other people involving himself multiply their happy lucky feeling under a difficult condition. Such a man has flexible and firm abdomen, grows younger, has good complexion and has the beautiful fire and power within his abdomen. In addition, following body-response, a powerful man, wise man or patient man can erase his unhappy feeling, multiply his happy lucky feeling or recover from disease under a difficult condition. Such a man can be called a efficient manager, too". It is such a man that is described for a sheepherder in the Scriptures. By the way, are you a powerful man, wise man, patient man, statesman, efficient manager or good sheepherder for you, your family, your friends or society?

According to The Power of Silence by Mr.Carlos Castaneda, don Juan Matus said "When we feel worthless, we should be fighting, not apologizing or feeling sorry for ourselves, and that it does not matter what our specific fate is as long as we face it with ultimate abandon".

"The new seers used petty tyrants not only to get rid of their self-importance, but to accomplish the very sophisticated maneuver of moving themselves out of this world" (The Fire From Within).

Subject:    How to good-by depression 10
From:       Hiroyuki Nishigaki
Date:       2000/01/01
Message-ID:
Newsgroups: depression
[More Headers]

Hello

## Writing about a petty tyrant touches me on a sore place

While I am writing about a petty tyrant, the parable of a petty tyrant touches me on a sore place. As for me, the complaint about my parents, the old bitter trouble, the pangs of spine, the stiff lamp of my underbelly, and my frequent urination had been a petty tyrant for about 20 years. Such a petty tyrant had made me irritated. Such a petty tyrant had made me have a terrible temper. I had sometimes lost my temper with my 3 daughters, a son, and my wife, and outrage them. I had been neither a good father nor a good husband. I had nearly become a new petty tyrant for them. I had been nearly defeated by my petty tyrant, but I had barely overcome it 2 years ago.

My petty tyrant had nearly deprived me of happy lucky feeling (power) such as peace, sweetness, cunning, joy, clarity, inner silence and flexibility. My eyes, my voice and my behavior had nearly lost happy lucky feeling for long years. My petty tyrant had made my immaterial fiber or third attention almost dead or useless so that my petty tyrant had made me become almost a blockhead for about 20 years.

If I had been weak or impatient, I had died of bladder cancer or high blood pressure. My petty tyrant of about 20 years had kept on torturing, weakening and trying to kill me, but it had fairly given me the attributes of a warrior which are control, discipline, forbearance, timing while I was barely fighting against my petty tyrant. Such a petty tyrant had been both an enemy and a benefactor for me.

Don Juan Matus (Mr. Carlos Castaneda's teacher) was a Yaqui Indian and had been much persecuted by Conquest. His parents were killed by Conquest. But, he looked younger and more energetic than his son, Ignacio Flores who was in his mid-sixties. His son still had the bearing of a military man (The Active Side of Infinity by Carlos Castaneda). I think don Juan Matus is stronger than me and the late Mr. Carlos Casteneda, because don Juan Matus had been confronted with much bigger petty tyrants than we had been confronted with, and had overcome them. Don Juan Matus had tempered himself owing to much bigger tyrants. The late Mr. Carlos Castaneda had accomplished a great achievement to write good books. But, I think the late Mr. Carlos Castaneda could not become a successor to don Juan Matus because he seemed to neither been confronted with a much bigger tyrant nor overcome it.

Hiroyuki Nishigaki<br>Spirit bless you!

Subject:    How to good-by depression 11
From:       Hiroyuki Nishigaki
Date:       2000/01/03
Message-ID:
Newsgroups: depression

A teacher, a Reverend or a guru have talked about such a light (fire) and asked for it for long years. Ironically, they seldom seems to have such a light in their abdomens. As a result, they are apt to have bad complexion, not to grow younger, not to become vigorous. Then, they are apt to die of cancer or heart disease. There are hundreds of ways to burn the fire from within our bodies. That is to say, there are hundreds of ways to temper your body and heart. They are like a maze. Most of us and even a teacher, a Reverend or (or not practicing everyday patiently, carefully, not-proudly and soberly).

I know many ways to temper my body and heart, so I am careful not to rove from one way to another and end up practicing no way the same as we rove from one woman(or man) to another woman(or man) and end up marrying with no woman(or no man) or bad woman(or man). If you do such a strange exercise, can confirm the effect in a few months and like it, you had better not have an affair with other exercises.

According to some German doctor, three biggest causes of cancer are unhappy childhood, keeping own feelings under and suffering from the stress of complaints (against an opposite sex, son or daughter, parents, money, work or post and so on) for more than 3 years. If you have not practiced some way to burn the fire from within, these causes can make the fire of your abdomen go out so that you have lost joy, become cynical. As a result, your body can not emit strong beautiful energy so that you have bad complexion, look older and have colder sticky numb part of your body. Cancer prefers only colder sticky numb part of your body and grows there. Or you may begin to suffer from depression.

It is much more effective to burn the fire from within your body that you know only 1-2 ways and keep on practicing it everyday for 10-20 years the same as the above mentioned 70 year old man does. I think you will neither die of cancer nor suffer from depression as long as you keep on burning the fire from within your body so that you have good complexion, grow at least 10-20 years younger and become vigorous.

Most readers may begin to practice the same way everyday after they read my contributions. But, I think most readers will stop practicing it in 2-3 months at the latest.

Hiroyuki Nishigaki

Spirit bless you!

Subject:    Re: How to good-by depression 11
From:       Hiroyuki Nishigaki
Date:       2000/01/04
Message-ID:
Newsgroups: depression
[More Headers]

Hi Lms

Subject:    Re: If you're planning to constrict your anus 2000 times…
From:       Lms
Date:       1999/12/21

We have our own university?!? Cool!
Q: How many feel like Ph.D's already?
Q: What would the course catalogue look like?
Liberal arts-To make our bodies stronger and healthier, we had better follow the life-style of long-living British people. Some news reported on the research on the life-style of about 7000 long-living British citizens about 10 years ago. The most contributing factors to their longevity, it was reported, were, to;
    1. Sleep daily for 7 hours
    2. Eat breakfast, lunch and dinner at regular hour
    3. Eat a well-balanced nutritious breakfast

4. Don't smoke

5.Don't drink alcohol whenever you want to stop

6.Maintain the standard weight of body

7.Practice proper body-exercise twice a week (for example, I recommend daily practicing of simple 5 Tibetan exercises as described in Ancient Secret of The Fountain of Youth, or the ancient Inca-style movement called Tensegrity) or walk for more than one hour everyday.

Those who practice all these 7 factors can live 10 years longer than those who follow only 6 of them. Those who follow all 7 of them can live 20 years longer than those who do not follow at all.

I think that such liberal arts are much more essential to fight against and overcome a petty tyrant which is the cause of depression and of cancer.

Without them, other exercises, preventions and medical treatments are useless.

By the way, most of us have to enter The University of Depression in our thirties or forties because of the complaint about opposite sex, parents, boss, money, work or post. After graduating from it, most of us have to enter The Graduate School of Depression after the age of 50 because of the death of spouse, divorce, big lost love, trouble about son or daughter, or loss of health, money, work, post.

It is very difficult for us to graduate from The Graduate School of Depression.If we can graduate from it, we will be able to live longer than the age of 80.

We already have a student union, right here!

Oh, and James? May I be excused from finals? I've got depression.

Don't lets fail the test!

—Lms

On 21 Dec 1999 19:02:42 GMT, Hiroyuki Nishigaki wrote:

Hello

Maybe, we do not have to peep into or play in the news-group of depression. We may graduate from The University of Depression. Don't let's fail the test.

From some snipped stuff.

Hiroyuki Nishigaki
Spirit bless you!

From:    Lms
Date:    Tue, 21 December 19999 02:18 PM EST

I nominate Mary Beth to lead the pep Squad.
GOOOO DEPRESSIONS!!!!!! feh....

Lms

Subject:    Re: If you're planning to constrict your anus 2000 times...
From:    Stob
Date:    1999/12/21
Message-ID:
Newsgroups: depression
[More Headers]

That one was pretty bad...but it reminds me of one of my new favorite jokes...I'll post it in a minute...

—-Stob

"That which does not kill me only makes me...stranger."

Hiroyuki Nishigaki
Spirit bless you!

Hello

Subject:   Re: How to good-by depression 11
From:      Aawa
Date:      Tue, 04 January 2000 01:59 PM EST
Message-id:

On 04 Jan 2000 12:03:05 GMT, Hiroyuki Nishigaki wrote:

Hi Lms


Subject:   Re: If you're planning to constrict your anus 2000 times...
From:      Lms
Date:      1999/12/21

We have our own university?!? Cool!

Q: How many feel like Ph.D's already?

Q: What would the course catalogue look like?

Liberal arts-To make our bodies stronger and healthier, we had better follow the life-style of long-living British people. Some news reported on the research on the life-style of about 7000 long-living British citizens about 10 years ago. The most contributing factors to their longevity, it was reported, were, to;

Damn, it's like a ghost from the past, I'm sad reading this.

It's all so absurd, I want to laugh, to cry, to scream, to constrict my anus and dent my navel all at the same time...ahh well.

Aawa

—Toto...I don't think we're in Kansas anymore.

Subject:    please, send me the poem
From:       Hiroyuki Nishigaki
Date:       2000/01/06
Message-ID:
Newsgroups: depression
[More Headers]

Hi

I am the writer of How to good-by depression (for example, constricting anus 100 times)in the newsgroup of depression. Someone, please, teach me the famous American poem whose title is Youth(the spring time of life) in English because I want to write about it in How to good-by depression. I can not translate it into English correctly because I am a foreigner.

Youth is not the period of life but the condition of heart...

Hiroyuki Nishigaki
Spirit bless you!

Subject:    Re: please, send me the poem
From:       Vwom
Date:       Thu, 06 January 2000 02:54 AM EST
Message-id:

On 06 Jan 2000 07:16:51 GMT, Hiroyuki Nishigaki said:

Hi

I am the writer of How to good-by depression (for example, constricting anus 100 times)in the newsgroup of. depression. Someone, please, teach me the famous American poem whose title is Youth(the spring time of life) in English because I want to write about it in How to good-by depression. I can not translate it into English correctly because I am a foreigner.

Youth is not the period of life but the condition of heart...

I found an English version here (scroll down towards the bottom):

http://www.mks.or.jp/...

—

doin' the low-carb, weight-lifting thang

# Part 3 Do 3-week fasting, save sex energy and rotate vortex

**Do 3-week fasting**

Subject:    How to good-by depression 12
From:       Hiroyuki Nishigaki
Date:       Thu, 06 January 2000 10:47 PM EST
Message-id:

Hi

3 week fasting can make you excrete a bucket of old black excrement (4-5 kg) and make your bowel movement regular.

To strengthen heart, you had better imagine self-confident, active, sexy, good-natured youth or women, eat bitter foods and massage the thumb's root of your left wrist.

The gates of heart is a small intestine and pancreas. So, you had better strengthen a small intestine and pancreas to strengthen heart, too. To strengthen a small intestine and pancreas, you had better make bowel movement regular. To make bowel movement regular, you had better feel hungry by moving your body well everyday and not eating too much. You had better become a vegetarian as possible. Furthermore, to bowel movement regular, you had better practice fasting for 3 weeks under the supervision of professional when you change job, are fired, retire or divorce.

Beautiful red part of below eyes is a evidence of recovering strong heart.

While practicing 3 week fasting, you can excrete a bucket of old black Excrement (4-5 kg) in your intestine. You become so relieved and happy that you feel as if you swept a foul chimney. The first day you excrete your old black excrement, the part just below your eyes will turn to be beautiful red.

Acridity, dreariness, self-pity will be removed from your eyes, too. The beautiful red part of your complexion is a evidence of recovering strong heart(in such a case, it is difficult for cancer to happen to you). Self-confidence and joy will happen to you naturally when beautiful strong red energy of your heart can burns violently again and can be shot out from your body like a flame of a flame-thrower and can swallow up an outside object. You can understand that self-pity will happen to you when red energy of your heart can not do so because your heart is beaten by the stickiness of your dirty energy, of other dirty energy, of devils, of your complaints(about health, opposite sex, son or daughter, parents, money, work, or post), can't you?

Your gunshot of * * will become longer than that of your high school for 2 weeks after finishing 3 week fasting. You will be able to take back Youth again. I think you will regret "I am stupid enough to have postponed practicing fasting till now".

My dear friend, a surgeon who runs a surgery hospital recommended me to do so 30 years ago. I practiced 3-week fasting 20 years ago for the first time. Since then, I have practiced 3 week fasting 5 times.

I think medical treatment is not enough to cure depression or cancer. So, I have neither taken the medicine of antidepressant nor gone to therapists even though I might suffer from depression because of a petty tyrant who is the cause of depression and of cancer. Furthermore, I will take neither the medical treatment nor operation if I am beaten by a petty tyrant and suffer from cancer. In such a case, I want to die while working or walking. I want to die not like an animal in a safe zoo but like a wild animal in a dangerous Africa plain.

Following such a thought, I am writing How to good-by depression series (or this book). I hope the readers who agree to my thought will only take advantage of some part of How to good-by depression series (or this book) at your peril.

Hiroyuki Nishigaki
Spirit bless you!


Subject:    Re: How to good-by depression 12
From:       Hiroyuki Nishigaki
Date:       Fri, 07 January 2000 05:08 AM EST
Message-id:

Hi Abea

I can begin to write about the way to cure constipation at last. Please, read it if you are interested in. I wish I could graduate from the subject about anus gradually. But I will not be able to do so for some time.


Subject:    Re: To constrict anus is Yoga way, too
From:       Abea
Date:       1999/12/18 01:20 PM EST
Message-ID:
Newsgroups: depression
[More Headers]

Damn. I always seem to get everything backwards! For all these years, I've been constricting my navel, and denting my anus. No wonder I'm constipated and depressed!

Abea


Subject:    Re: To constrict anus is Yoga way, too
From:       Hiroyuki Nishigaki
Date:       1999/12/19 GMT
Message-ID:
Newsgroups: depression
[More Headers]

Hello Abea

To cure constipation is essential to cure depression. I will wrote about it in How to good-by depression 4-6. So, please, wait for a while. I had had the bad bowel movement, but I can go to stool a few times everyday now.


Subject:    Re: To constrict anus is Yoga way, too
From:       Aawa
Date:       Sat, 18 December 1999 10:01 PM EST
Message-ID:
Newsgroups: depression

On 19 Dec 1999 02:30:51 GMT,Hiroyuki Nishigaki wrote:

Hello Abea

To cure constipation is essential to cure depression. I will wrote about it in How to good-by depression 4-6. So, please, wait for a while. I had had the bad bowel movement, but I can go to stool a few times everyday now.

What is this Crap?

Aawa

Toto I don't think we're in Kansas anymore

Subject:   Re: To constrict anus is Yoga way, too
From:      Abea
Date:      Sat, 18 December 1999 10:17 PM EST
Message-ID:
Newsgroups: depression

This is freakin' priceless!
ROFL!!!

Abea
Hiroyuki Nishigaki
Spirit bless you!

Subject:   Re: How to good-by depression 12
From:      Aah
Date:      Thu, 13 January 2000 10:57 AM EST
Message-id:

In article, Hiroyuki Nishigaki writes

3 week fasting can make you excrete a bucketful of old black excrement(4-5 kg) and make your bowel movement regular.

Why does this make me feel better about my tooth?
—

Aah~~~~~~~~~~~~~~~~~~~~~~~~~~~~~~~~~~~~~~~~~~~~~~~~
~~~~~~~~~~~~~~~~~~~~~~~~~~~~~~~~

The opinions given above may be mine. They might also just be what I feel like saying right now, okay?

Subject:   Re: How to good-by depression 12
From:      Rsuz
Date:      2000/01/14
Message-ID:
Newsgroups: depression
[More Headers]

I don't recommend eating dinner while reading this!
This is funny

Subject:   Re: How to good-by depression 12
From:      Hiroyuki Nishigaki
Date:      Sun, 23 January 2000 11:29 PM EST
Message-id:

Dear Aah
Such a response is called body-response. Your body-response
has special meaning for you. You have to solve it for yourself.
Body response happens when we can feel happy or healthy, have
good complexion and do not get stuck or depressed.

Subject:   Re: How to good-by depression 12
From:      Aah
Date:      Thu, 13 January 2000 10:57 AM EST
Message-id:

In article, Hiroyuki Nishigaki writes

3 week fasting can make you excrete a bucket of old black
excrement (4-5 kg) and make your bowel movement regular.
Why does this make me feel better about my tooth?

Hiroyuki Nishigaki

URL http://hometown.aol.com/hnishigaki/index.htm
Spirit bless you!


Subject:   How to good-by depression 13
From:      Hiroyuki Nishigaki
Date:      Sun, 09 January 2000 06:36 AM EST
Message-id:

Hello

Those who enter a center of fasting are apt to talk about delicious foods and old black excrement which has stuck to their small intestine for long years while staying for 3 weeks at a center of fasting.

If you enter a center of fasting, you will have to stop drinking alcohol and coffee, stop smoking, stop being on meds, stop making love, stop eating animal food, animal-protein and white sugar.

You have to keep on decreasing the amount of foods by one-seventh everyday for a first week. After a first week you will have to drink only water everyday for a second week. After a second week you will have to begin to eat again little by little everyday for a third week. For a third week you will have to keep on increasing the amount of foods by one-seventh everyday. Then, You will leave a center of fasting and be able to eat the ordinary amount of foods. For a fourth and a fifth week, you had better stop drinking alcohol and coffee, stop smoking, stop being on meds, stop eating animal food, animal-protein and white sugar.

For a first week and a third week you have to chew every mouthful of food 200 times when you eat foods. You have to drink water without chlorine every 30 minutes in the daytime for 3 weeks at a center of fasting. If you can not drink natural water, you have to pour water with chlorine into a big bowl, leave it for a day and make chlorine evaporate from water. Next day you can drink water without chlorine. Furthermore, you have to take one-hour stroll and do one hour proper body exercise everyday at a center of fasting.

While staying at a center of fasting, you have to make every effort to do bowel movement everyday. If you can not do bowel movement everyday, you have to do so with the help of laxative or enema.

Your old black excrement which has stuck to your small intestine for long years will begin to be excreted from a fourth day you begin to drink only water at a center of fasting or by a week later you leave a center of fasting. Just before you begin to excrete old black excrement for the first time, you will feel abdominal pains more or less. Your small intestine may bleed.

If you practice 3 week fasting, you can lose weight by 8-10 kg. You will lose weight by net 4-5 kg because you have excreted a bucket of old black excrement(4-5 kg) in your intestine. You become so relieved and happy that you feel as if you swept a foul chimney. The first day you excrete your old black excrement, the part just below your eyes will turn to be beautiful red.

Acridity, dreariness, self-pity will be removed from your eyes, too. The beautiful red part of your complexion is a evidence of recovering strong heart ( in such a case, it is difficult for cancer to happen to you).

Strong heart is the cause of self-confidence and of joy. Self-confidence and joy will happen to you naturally when beautiful strong red energy of your heart can burns violently again and can be shot out from your body like a flame of a flame-thrower and can swallow up an outside object.

You can understand that self-pity will happen to you when red energy of your heart can not do so because your heart is beaten by the stickiness of your dirty energy, of other dirty energy, of devils, of your complaints( about health, opposite sex, son or daughter, parents, money, work, or post), can't you?

Your gunshot of * * will become longer than that of your high school for 2 weeks after finishing 3 week fasting. You will be able to take back Youth again. I think you will regret? I am stupid enough to have postponed practicing fasting till now.?

You will be able to enjoy happy lucky feeling like that of Ulman's poem for the first time. I imagine you may weep because the injury of your heart has been healed by 3 week fasting.

"YOUTH"

Youth is not a time of life? it is a state of mind; it is a temper of the will, a quality of the imagination, a vigor of the emotions, a predominance of courage over timidity, of the appetite for adventure over love of ease.

Nobody grows old by merely living a number of years; people grow old only by deserting their ideals. Years wrinkle the skin, but to give up enthusiasm wrinkles the soul. Worry, doubt, self-distrust, fear and despair—these are the long, long years that bow the head and turn the growing spirit to back to dust.

Whether seventy or sixteen, there is in every being's heart the love of wonder, the sweet amazement at the stars and the starlike things and thoughts, the undaunted challenge of events, the unfailing childlike appetite for what next, and the joy and the game of life.

You are as young as your faith, as old as your doubt; as young as your self-confidence, as old as your fear, as young as your hope, as old as your despair.

So long as your heart receives messages of beauty, cheer, courage, grandeur and power from the earth, from man and from the Infinite, so long you are young.

When the wires are all down and all the central place of your heart is covered with the snows of pessimism and the ice of cynicism, then you are grown old indeed and may God have mercy on your soul.

By Ulman, an American poet

I hope someone who has practiced 3 week fasting at least three times for 10 years will post a contribution about 3 week fasting (or someone who has kept on doing some proper exercise everyday for 10 years following the life style of long-lived British as possible or can turn to bay throwing away pride ) to How to good-by depression. But, I think it is almost impossible because someone who has practiced 3 week fasting at least three times for 10 years (or someone who has kept on doing some proper exercise everyday for 10 years or can turn to bay throwing away pride) does not need to peep into the news group of depression.

Some reader may wonder why I peep into the news group of depression although I have practiced 3 week fasting 6 times for 20 years. It is because I have been fighting against a petty tyrant who is the cause of depression and of cancer. At some time I might have been diagnosed as depression or bladder cancer if I had gone to doctors. I can have survived without medical treatment or meds. As a result, I have a friendly feeling to the reader or contributors of the newsgroup of depression and have played the part of snipped staff.

Hiroyuki Nishigaki
Spirit bless you!

Subject:    Re: How to good-by depression 13
From:       Lmou
Date:       Sun, 09 January 2000 09:38 AM EST
Message-id:

What on earth do these people come from???

Lmou

On 09 Jan 2000 11:36:28 GMT, Hiroyuki Nishigaki wrote:

Hello

Those who enter a center of fasting are apt to talk about delicious foods and old black excrement which has stuck to their small intestine for long years while staying for 3 weeks at a center of fasting.

If you enter a center of fasting, you will have to stop drinking alcohol and coffee, stop smoking, stop being on meds, stop making love, stop eating animal food, animal-protein and white sugar.

You have to keep on decreasing the amount of foods by one-seventh everyday for a first week. After a first week you will have to drink only water everyday for a second week. After a second week you will have to begin to eat again little by little everyday for a third week. For a third week you will have to keep Then, You will leave a center of fasting and be able to eat the ordinary amount of foods.

For a fourth and a fifth week, you had better stop drinking alcohol and coffee, stop smoking, stop being on meds, stop eating animal food, animal-protein and white sugar.

For a first week and a third week you have to chew every mouthful of food 200 times when you eat foods.

You have to drink a cup of natural water or water without chlorine every 30 minutes in the daytime for 3 weeks at a center of fasting. If you can not drink natural water, you have to pour water with chlorine into a big bowl, leave it for a day and make chlorine evaporate from water Next day you can drink water without chlorine. Furthermore, you have to take one-hour stroll and do one hour proper body exercise every-day at a center of fasting.

While staying at a center of fasting, you have to make every effort to do bowel movement everyday. If you can not do bowel movement everyday, you have to do so with the help of laxative or enema.

Your old black excrement which has stuck to your small intestine for long years will begin to be excreted from a fourth day you begin to drink only water at a center of fasting or by a week later you leave a center of fasting. Just before you begin to excrete old black excrement for the first time, you will feel abdominal pains more or less. Your small intestine may bleed.

If you practice 3 week fasting, you can lose weight by 8-10 kg. You will lose weight by net 4-5 kg because you have excreted a bucket of old black excrement(4-5 kg) in your intestine. You become so relieved and happy that you feel as if you swept a foul chimney. The first day you excrete your old black excrement, the part just below your eyes will turn to be beautiful red.

Acridity, dreariness, self-pity will be removed from your eyes, too. The beautiful red part of your complexion is a evidence of recovering strong heart(in such a case, it is difficult for cancer to happen to you).

Strong heart is the cause of self-confidence and of joy. Self-confidence and joy will happen to you naturally when beautiful strong red energy of your heart can burns violently again and can be shot out from your body like a flame of a flame-thrower and can swallow up an outside object.

You can understand that self-pity will happen to you when red energy of your heart can not do so because your heart is beaten by the stickiness of your dirtyenergy, of other dirty energy, of devils, of your complaints( about health,opposite sex, son or daughter, parents, money, work, or post), can't you?

Your gunshot of **will become longer than that of your high school for 2 weeks after finishing 3 week fasting. You will be able to take back Youth I think you will regret "I am stupid enough to have postponed practicing fasting till now".

You will be able to enjoy happy lucky feeling like that of Ulman's poem for the first time. I imagine you may weep because the injury of your heart has been healed by 3 week fasting.

OUTH it is a state of mind; it is a temper of the will, a quality of the imagination, a vigor of the emotions, a predominance of courage over timidity, of the appetite for adventure over love of ease.

Nobody grows old by merely living a number of years; people grow old only by deserting their ideals. Years wrinkle the skin, but to give up enthusiasm wrinkles the soul. Worry, doubt, self-distrust, fear and despair—these are the long, long years that bow the head and turn the growing spirit to back to dust.

Whether seventy or sixteen, there is in every being's heart the love of wonder, the sweet amazement at the stars and the starlike things and thoughts, the undaunted challenge of events, the unfailing childlike appetite for what next, and the joy and the game of life.

You are as young as your faith, as old as your doubt; as young as your self-confidence, as old as your fear, as young as your hope, as old as your despair.

So long as your heart receives messages of beauty, cheer, courage, grandeur and power from the earth, from man and from the Infinite, so long you are young.

When the wires are all down and all the central place of your heart is covered with the snows of pessimism and the ice of cynicism, then you are grown old indeed and may God have mercy on your soul.

By Ulman, an American poet

I hope someone who has practiced 3 week fasting at least three times for 10 years will post a contribution about 3 week fasting(or someone who has kept on doing some proper exercise everyday for 10 years following the life style of long-lived British as possible or can turn to bay throwing away pride ) to How to good-by depression. But, I think it is almost impossible because someone who has practiced 3 week fasting at least three times for 10 years(or someone who has kept on doing some proper exercise everyday for 10 years following the life style of long-lived British as possible or can turn to bay throwing away pride ) does not need to peep into the newsgroup of depression.

Some reader may wonder why I peep into the newsgroup of depression although I have practiced 3 week fasting 6 times for 20 years. It is because I have been fighting against a petty tyrant which is the cause of depression and of cancer. At some time I might have been diagnosed as depression or bladder cancer if I had gone to doctors. I can have survived without medical treatment or meds. As a result, I have a friendly feeling to the reader or contributors of the newsgroup of depression and have played the part of snipped staff.

Hiroyuki Nishigaki
Spirit bless you!

"I'm all out of faith, this is how I feel"
"You'r a little late, I'm already torn"

Mni

Subject:　Re: How to good-by depression 13
From:　　Hiroyuki Nishigaki
Date:　　Mon, 10 January 2000 10:44 PM EST
Message-id:

Hello
It is effective way to strengthen and purify our energy that we will read the poem, Youth loudly for one hour twice a day every-day for more than 3 years. I think to read it loudly for 2 hours everyday for more than 3 years is effective to cure depression.

Hiroyuki Nishigaki
Spirit bless you!

How to good-by depression 14
When you enter a center of fasting, you have to deposit all of your money in a center of fasting. While doing 3-week fast-ing, you feel hungry very much. Furthermore, your nose becomes sensitive enough to catch the smell of every house's cooking while taking a stroll.

If you have money, hunger and sensitiveness of nose are apt to impel you to buy food and eat it or enter a restaurant and eat food. If you do so while doing 3-week fasting, you will die. Especially it is very dangerous that you eat something or eat extra food without chewing 200 times after a forth day of only drinking water and eating nothing.

Someone sometimes dies because he does not deposit all of his money in a center of fasting and buy food or enter a restaurant and eat food. While taking a stroll, I am often impelled to stop walking in front of some house and sniff the smell of some house's cooking. I can awake what dinner or lunch the family of some house will eat today. When I did a sixth 3-week fasting one and half an years ago, I was impelled to enter a bakery without having money and was on the brink of buy bread although I knew it is dangerous to eat food. I brought bread to the cash desk, then I awoke I could not buy it because I did not have money.

After you leave a center of fasting, you have to stop drinking alcohol and coffee, stop smoking, stop being on meds, stop eating animal food, animal-protein and white sugar for 2 weeks. A week later I left a center of fasting, I was impelled to drink a cup of coffee and felt much pain as if I drank oil. I groaned with pain on my bed all day for 2 days.

Furthermore, you have to be careful not to fall down in a faint like a log while doing 3-week fasting. If you leap up, you will fall down in a faint easily, so you have to stand up slowly. You had better squat as soon as you begin to fall down because of anemia while walking or standing. While doing a third 3-week fasting, I fell down in a faint like a log 4 times because of my conceit and carelessness. I fell down to a big stone once, but fortunately my teeth were not broken.

You feel the dullest and the most tired 4 days later you begin to eat nothing. It takes you twice more time to walk the same way. Then, strangely you will become energetic day by day.

When I did a sixth 3-week fasting and took one hour stroll one and half an years ago, I was much surprised that both of my legs fell into a fit of convulsions and could not walk at all. I was at a loss because I could not find a public phone. The road was narrow, so no taxi was running. It began to rain. Then, I suddenly remembered the right way of walking which Carlos Castaneda's teacher, don Juan Matus taught his disciplines. While walking, I curled my fingers of my hands, drew my attention to my arms, made the middle of my eyebrows broadened, made my view broadened to 180 degree and kept on looking at the horizon. Strangely I could cure the convulsions of my legs soon and walk smoothly.

After you leave a center of fasting, you have to be careful not to become fat because any food is more delicious than before. You had better not eat too much.

For 20 years I have done 3-week fasting 3 times at a center of fasting and done 3-week fasting 3 times working usually. I want to challenge 45-day fasting this year or next year.

How to good-by depression 15

If you want to enter a center of fasting, you have to stop taking the medicine, stop drinking alcohol, coffee, water with chlorine, stop smoking, by the kettle of aluminum everyday from 2 weeks or a month earlier before you enter it. If you do not follow it, you will feel much painful at a center of fasting. Especially you have to emit the toxin of medicine from your body as possible before you enter a center of fasting. The toxin of the medicine of adrenal cortex hormone is the most dangerous while you are doing 3-week fasting. It drills a hole in your stomach. It is difficult for you to enter it if you have taken the medicine of adrenal cortex hormone.

The toxin of the medicine, chlorine and the constituent parts of alcohol, of tabacco, of vinyl, of plastic, of aluminum and of favorite foods are discharged from the sweat gland of your skin, from your tongue and from the recess of your throat. They emit bad smell so that people who stay at a center of fasting and its rooms emit peculiar bad smell.

You have to scrub your skin with a wet towel many times everyday to prevent the sweat gland of your skin from getting stuck by such dirty excretions. Your tongue and the recess of your throat turn to be white and sticky. So, you have to often scrub off them with toothbrush. You have to stop making-up, stop using chemical soap and chemical toothpaste at a center of fasting.

You can feel that the peculiar happy lucky feeling will run away day by day after you leave a center of fasting and begin to break the rules of fasting. You may think it is the toxin of old black excrement, of medicine, of alcohol, of chlorine, of tabacco, of vinyl, of plastic, of aluminum and of favorite foods that is a petty tyrant or devil who keeps on weakening us, making us a blockhead and depriving us of light spring breeze's feeling, joy, abandon, largess, humor, instinct, inspiration, peace, sweet, clarity, kindness, bravery, patience and originality. I think they look like a web of a spider that catches us and deprives us of freedom.

While doing a sixth 3-week fasting one and half a years ago, I was surprised to awake that such a toxin within my body gathered to my medula oblongata. Medula oblongata is so important organ for us that we have to die soon if a needle sticks it. I felt as if such a toxin within our medula oblongata were like virus within a personal computer, too.

When you begin to eat and drink after you leave a center of fasting, you can awake to the smell of chlorine and of the constituent parts of vinyl, of plastic, of aluminum. You can awake that your sensory organ which has been revived and refreshed by 3 week fasting begin to be destroyed by the toxin of the medicine, chlorine and the constituent parts of alcohol, of tabacco, of vinyl, of plastic, of aluminum day by day. Your sensory organ has been revived and refreshed enough to understand a happy lucky feeling like that of Ulman poem. But….It is regrettable.

How to good-by depression 16

When I meet the men or women who try to persecute, anger, irritate or bother me to no end, I think the old black solid excrement of these people's small intestines make these people speak, think or act in such a way so that I will not get so angry.

The old 4-5 kg black solid excrement which has stuck to a small intestine for long year keeps on emitting toxin and circulating it all over body. As a result, it has made us weaken our hearts and livers and made us have bad complexion, bad bowel movement, bad appetite, bad sleeping, bad sex or stiff shoulder. Heart is the origin of joy, self-confidence and abandon. Liver is the origin of light spring breeze's feeling or tree sprouts' feeling.

Its toxin has weakened heart and liver so that it has deprived us of a peculiar happy lucky feeling such as joy, self-confidence, abandon, light spring breeze's feeling or tree sprouts' feeling. Furthermore, heart is connected with a small intestine by energy channel. If a small intestine has been weakened by a bucketful of the old black solid excrement, heart has lost beautiful strong red energy and joy, self-confidence. In such a case we are apt to have bad complexion and indulge in self-pity, worthlessness, stinginess, cowardice.

I think unhappy-unhealthy-inefficient people and founders, big men, pioneers, enterprisers who will become disgraced in 3-5 years (or 10 years or a year) are apt to become little petty tyrants or small-fry persecute or anger or bother other people to no end. They have bad complexion. They seem to have much old black excrement that has stuck to their small intestines for long years. They are not grateful but a grumbler. They are proud or careless. They take so many liberties.

When I meet the men or women who have bad complexion, have acrid, dreary or self-pity eyes, look older or take many liberties, I am apt to imagine that they have much old black solid excrement. Old black excrement is as solid as plastic. So, we have to drink a cup of water every 30 minutes everyday at a center of fasting to soften old black excrement.

If we can excrete the old black excrement which has much toxin, we will be able to begin to burn the fire from within our bodies, erase the bad stickiness of our bodies (which our complaint, dirties energy of others or devil has given us), erase our sad or hateful personal histories and strengthen our hearts and livers so that we will have good complexion, grow younger and enjoy a peculiar happy lucky feeling such as joy, self-confidence, abandon, light spring breeze's feeling or tree sprouts' feeling. When I took one-hour stroll while doing a first 3-week fasting about 20 years ago, a pillar of fire sometimes ascended to the inside of my head from my abdomen suddenly and I could awake the burning smell of fire within my head. I felt a little pain in the recesses of my nose. Tears ran down my face because of a pillar of fire.

If we have strengthen our heart, we can enjoy the same feeling as that of self-confident, joyful, active, sexy, ruthless, good-natured youth or women. Healthy strong heart has the red energy of such a feeling. Such a red energy can swallow up and burn our dirty energy (stickiness, the fever of depression, numbness and coldness), the dirty energy of other and devils. So, it can cure our diseases or others' diseases. If it is shot out from our body, it can keep on catching on an outside object, swallow up an object, and burn the bad energy of an object. Light dances wildly in front of our eyes just before such a red energy succeeds in swallowing up our dirty energy, the dirty energy of other, devils, and an outside object. Then, self-pity passes away. So, the feeling of self-confidence and of ruthlessness happen to us.

Regretfully, most of us have thrown away such a red energy after most of us have lost a big love, was divorced, betrayed, beaten, were raised in cold family or failed in something, too. As a result, most of us have lost beautiful glossy red color on our complexion or begun to have dirty black red color on our complexion. Stiff shoulder has happened, too. Most of us have become cynical, weak-minded, and stingy. Most of us prefer to gossips about other. Most of us hate taking care of other. At last, horizontal line has begun to be seen between eyes and a strange feeling (a little pain, numbness, or impotence) has begun to happen to a little finger. Many red spots have happened to the back of neck. At last, cardiac infarction, angina pectoris, or cancer will happen sooner or later.

If you have strengthen your liver, you can enjoy the same good feeling as that of light spring breeze, of a tree's sprout or of an innocent adolescent. Most of us have thrown away such a feeling since most of us begin to have the trouble of spine or some complaints about opposite sex, health, son or daughter, parents, boss, money, work or post. I had forgotten such a feeling for about 40 years, too. Sometimes, I can have begun to enjoy such a feeling since 2 years ago. I feel as if light spring breeze skimmed through my body. Then, I am engulfed by beautiful blue or green energy. I feel as if I have revived.

Blue energy is like the feeling of light spring breeze, of a tree's sprout or of an innocent adolescent. Blue energy has a special power. It seems to be weak at first, but it is really strong. It can make others relaxed and revived. It has a peculiar pheromone. It can disarm anybody without orders or threat, and can use anybody freely without order or money. Anybody is apt to follow it voluntarily. It is apt to gain, use, and control anybody or anything without endeavor to do so. If big men, founders, pioneers or enterpriser weaken their livers and lose the feeling of light spring breeze, they will be disgraced miserably by the attacks of many other people because they only use stick and do not give carrot to other people.

Most of us have thrown away such a strange blue energy after most of us lost a big love, were divorced, betrayed, beaten, were raised in cold family or failed in something. If we have thrown away it, we will become like machines without lubricant. We will lose cunning and smooth. Unhappy-unhealthy-inefficient people lack in such a strange blue energy. As a result, they will become dull, tired, or irritated. They will lack in sex energy that has a close connection with liver. They can make ** with opposite sex only once or twice a month even if they want to do so more times. They may have a terrible temper, too. They think "I can not believe other people. I have to depend upon only myself". They become cynical. Then, they become like inefficient machines without lubricant, so that they will be able to neither believe other people nor depend upon themselves after all. They will be able to believe neither other people nor themselves, so that they will become more cynical and will not recover light spring breeze's feeling of blue energy for long years or forever.

Happy-healthy-efficient people or big men have such a blue strange energy more or less which seduce other people. So, we have to endeavor not to throw away such a strange blue energy when we fail in something.

I flow such a strange blue energy to someone in secret when I am full of such a strange blue energy. Then, someone will send me a present or call to invite me even though I do not ask to do so.

In most cases, such a happy lucky feeling as that of Ulman poem-Youth will pass away 2 weeks later after you left a center of fasting. You will begin to eat animal food, animal-protein, much sugar, much salt, take the medicine, drink coffee, alcohol, smoke, do not chew well, do not have a stroll, do not do some proper exercise everyday, make ** with opposite sex, waste much sex energy so that happy relieved feeling will pass away. Needless to say, the gunshot of our **will become short again.

But, I think it is very important that we can have remembered, understood and recognized with the help of 3-week fasting what a happy lucky feeling of Youth is. Most of us have forgotten such a happy lucky feeling completely for long years since most of us were raised in cold family, lost a big love, divorced, were betrayed or complained about spouse, parents, son or daughter, boss, money, work or post.

You can understand what the aim is owing to doing 3-week fasting. To achieve the aim to take back such a happy lucky feeling as that of Ulman's poem, Youth, we had better keep on constricting anus 100 times in succession and denting navel 100 times in succession after constricting anus 100 times in succession everyday with satisfaction everyday following the life style of long-lived British everyday as possible.

If you constrict anus 100 times in succession and dent navel 100 times in succession after constricting anus 100 times in succession everyday, you will begin to feel a peculiar happy lucky feeling little by little in a month or a few month. Then, you will begin to have good complexion, and begin to talk, look at or act with abandon, largess, and humor. You will become more charming without make-up. As a result, you will begin to be asked by many other people "You have changed. You begin to have good complexion and your eyes are twinkling. Has anything good happened to you recently?". You may reply "Because I read some book, and I have tried at my peril" or you may simply smile secretively. If you are a woman, you will begin to be more loved by your husband or be made a proposal by many men.

### Save sex energy if possible

In addition your sex energy will begin to become strong again by constricting anus 100 times and denting navel 100 times everyday following the life style of long lived British. But, you had better reduce the frequency of **and of ## to less then half If possible

If you are less than 40 or 50 years old, you may become impatient and want to rape secretively. You will not be able to sleep thirsting for a young beautiful woman or man almost all night at the beginning. You feel something strong is about to pierce through the center of your body. When you live in moderation and regularity, practicing physical excise and saving your sex energy, something positive must happen to you sooner or later.

Surprisingly, you are not tired in spite of little sleep and start beginning to feel happier. If you eat sea vegetable as well everyday, your hair will grow back blond or black in 2-3 months. Hair may even start growing where on balding areas. The same as that of name card in water of a cup. Next day you eat it and drink this water. I was much surprised that my hair grew back black. I could not believed, so I pulled about ten white hairs of my head a few times for a month. I could confirm that my white hairs began to grow back black from their roots. Also your complexion changes for better and you grow younger. Your eyes begin to twinkle. Gray hair of head-white hair of face-white hair of **-white hair of ##-pass away. "here do you have gray hair on your body now?".

You'll be very pleased to realize to become full of energy for the first time. Within a year, some part of your body may become painful, hot, and may shiver. Then, the root chakra between anus and sexual organ, anus, or sexual organ sometimes may begin to shoot out energy violently like a big blank.

Such a big blank is much more violent than nocturnal emission, diarrhea and **. You look into your brief secretively. You brief is not wet or dirty, so you are very pleased to realize to become full of energy for the first time. That is to say, you have had strong immaterial fibers of root chakra, anus, or sexual organ that shoot out downwards or diagonally at last.

By these strong immaterial fibers, you can please the opposite sex more than before. But, you better save your sex energy as much as possible if you want to feel much happier, become healthier or more instinctive, and increase your supernatural power. The degree of your supernatural power is in proportion to the degree of your sex energy, of your beautiful strong fire within your abdomen, of your happy feeling, of your health, of your inner silence, of your good complexion, of your good bowel movement, of your instinct, of your rejuvenation, of your strength, of your nimbleness, of your flexibility, of your subtle breathing, and of your energy body's beauty[dryness, cool, sweet, fluidity].

Strong full sex energy can get up to warm the core of abdomen within the central energy pipe of your body. Then, the fire begins to burn within the core of abdomen. At the beginning, the fire suddenly rises from the core of abdomen to swallow you so that you are swallowed by red energy and can not see besides it for a while. Since then, you can often feel and see the fire suddenly rises within your central energy pipe. When you look into your body, you see the fire is burning from within your body.

Happy, healthy or successful people have strong sex energy, and beautiful strong immaterial fire within their abdomen and supernatural power. Ironically, most pastors and most teachers of the psychic world are apt to have bad complexion, weakness and solidity, and look old. Their believers often have better complexion, more strength and flexibility, grow younger, and look happier than most pastors and psychic teachers.

Ironically, unhappy people, who need supernatural power to become happy or healthy, have not supernatural power at all. Happy people, who do not need supernatural power to become happier than now, have much supernatural power. In this respect, unhappy people are apt not to be able to understand my writings at all. Happy, healthy, or successful people can understand my writings easily and will agree with it.

For example, happy, healthy, or successful people have strong sex energy and beautiful immaterial fire within their bodies, too. It is such a fire that is the medicine to cure or prevent depression. Furthermore, such a fire is the origin of supernatural power, of happiness, of health, of successful concentration, of success, of erasing the bad stickiness of our bodies, of rotating the vortex of our bodies, of shooting immaterial fibers or third attention to an outside object from our bodies, of rejuvenation, of good complexion, of good bowel movement, of instinct, of subtle breath, of strength, of flexibility or of seer. It is effective to turn on such a fire that we keep on constricting anus 100 times in succession and denting navel 100 times in succession after constricting anus 100 times in succession everyday for more than 10 years or at least a few years.

Besides shooting out a big blank from your buttock, you can feel as if your root chakra leaked sweet hot mucus. You can feel your root chakra as if it were a exciting womb. Cabala says "human being could have lived on the earth of high temperature long years ago as a human being of immaterial hermaphrodite". I think there has been the imprint of immaterial hermaphrodite in our physical body.

An about 30 year old man, who has a wife, has kept on constricting anus 100 times in succession and denting navel 100 times in succession after constricting anus 100 times in succession everyday following the life style of long-lived British as possible since January 1998. He can begin to spend winter, even in snow or outdoor with a short-sleeved although he has low blood pressure, not higher than 90.

I went skiing with him just after he completed 2-week fasting in winter in 1999. He said he felt as if he had beaten the earth with his legs, and the white spirit engulfed him for the first time while skiing.

You may beat the earth with your legs or hands as if the earth were a drum. Your strong energy shoots out into the earth and the earth begins to shiver whenever you beat the earth. When you can beat the earth, the earth looks like a gassy big ball or something fluid.

After such a phenomenon, a big explosion will begin to occur within your head, chest, abdomen, or legs. My first big explosion occurred within my head during the flight by plane over the Arctic Circle. When a big explosion occurred within abdomen one and half a years ago, I felt dizzy and could not stand up for a while. Your abdomen may begin to shoot out a big blank upward through the top of your head, and a big vortex of your energy may begin to whirl automatically within your head, chest, abdomen or legs.

Energetic vortexes of our bodies have been called a dragon in China. There are two types of vortexes. Automatically, one rotates horizontally within the physical body, another rotates vertically on the surface of physical body or within physical body.

The vortex begins to rotate automatically within physical body horizontally or vertically after a big explosion occurs within the head, chest, abdomen, or legs and central energy pipe between the root chakra of buttock and the crown chakra of head begins to be cleaned up. I asked the previously mentioned man who has kept on constricting anus 100 times in succession and denting navel 100 times in succession after constricting anus 100 times in succession everyday following the life style of long-lived British as possible since January 1998 and who has become so vigorous that he can begin to spend winter, even in snow or outdoors with short-sleeved "Can a big explosion occur or Can your vortex begin to rotate automatically, because you have become so vigorous that you can spend cold this winter with half-sleeved?".He replied "None of them has happened to me". I said "very strange. Why? ""I can understand the origin. It is because you are very intimate with your wife". He replied "I am not so intimate with my wife". I said "much more strange. Why? Why?".

He replied "I have done [] []" reluctantly. So, I said "You had better reduce the frequency of [] []"to less than half, and the rotation of your vortexes and a big explosion will happen to you in a year or 2 years as long as you keep on constricting anus 100 times in succession and denting navel 100 times in succession after constricting anus 100 times in succession everyday following the life style of long-lived British every day as possible saving your sex energy".

In my first manuscript of this book, I had not written it to respect his private life. But, I think saving your sex energy as much as possible is the indispensable step for you to be able to become healthier, feel happier or accomplish something special. So, I dare add it.

The secret of big men's is having strong living vortexes that rotate and work on.

Besides the vortex of your abdomen, other strong living vortexes of your physical body can shoot out immaterial strong fibers or the third attention to an outside object from your body and judge-control it. Strong living vortexes of your abdomen and of other parts of your physical body can send orders, messages, sounds, colors, smells, emotion, attack, or healing power to other people, animals, plants, trees or stars with these carried on the immaterial fiber or on the third attention. In such a case, your immaterial fiber or third attention is not confined to your body but shoots out to an outside object, catch it and control it. Furthermore, you can receive inspiration and power from an outside object. This is concentration indeed. That is to say, you can succeed in concentrating on something. Then, You can feel a much more happy lucky feeling, feel relieved and relaxed, feel self-confidence and soften your stiff shoulder so that you will cure or prevent depression, have better complexion, have better bowel movement, grow much younger, have stronger sex energy, become more healthy, attract many good healthy people, have more supernatural power and become more efficient.

That is to say, big men or those who have accomplished something, lived longer, grown more than 10-20 years younger, been happy, healthy, or been liked by many of the opposite sex, have good strong living vortexes which rotate and work on and can shoot out immaterial fibers or third attention to other people, animal, tree, flower, nature, sun, moon, stars, sports or hobby. That is to say, the cause of misunderstanding, illusion, failure, depression, disease, unhappiness, self-pity or inefficiency is to have much dirty stickiness, make body's fire go out, have bad complexion, be unable to rotate the vortex of body, be unable to shoot out immaterial fiber or third attention to an outside object, be unable to concentrate on it, be unable to judge it accurately and be unable to control or change it. The patriarch of Chinese Taoism says "One is wise who recognizes oneself as a stupid". But sometimes, I feel so regretful that I recognize I lived in so-called hell for most of my life because my vortexes have barely begun to rotate automatically since the age of 50, shoot out my immaterial fiber or third attention to an outside object and concentrate on it. Strangely, even the vortex on the surface of my chin sometimes rotates automatically.

Complaints(about opposite sex, son or daughter, parents, boss, money, work or post), other dirty energy bodies, devils, and the floating immaterial above your head are giving you dirtiness, stickiness, fever, coldness, solidity, or numbness which can weaken you so as to kill you. If you have big some complaint or If dirty energy bodies and devils often visit your vortex on the surface of your body or within your body or stick to your body for a long time, your vortex will begin to rotate under groan the same as the fan rotates within sewage, sink, or mud. Furthermore, your aura around you, energy channel of your internal organ, and your internal organ will become like sewage, sink or mud. As a result, more dirty energy bodies of others' and more devils will visit or stick to your vortex, energy channel, or internal organ, such as vultures, hyenas, or maggots.

The dirty, sticky, feverish, cold or solid immaterial[which is almost the world of the animal killed by you mercilessly and unnecessarily]begins to be floating above your head and your house, or around you, too. It is always connected with you through strong sticky wet immaterial pipe. Through this pipe, it can always run the dirty, sticky, feverish, cold or solid immaterial into you which can weaken or torture you. If you want to cure your or other's disease, you have to be able to see this strong sticky wet immaterial pipe such as a strong floating anchor, cut it, and set yourself or others free.

Because of your bigger complaint, of more attacks by dirty energy bodies, devils or of the floating dirty, sticky, feverish, cold or solid immaterial, your vortex becomes such as a fan in cold heavy oil, sludge, coal tar, cold clay, or solid snot. Then, your vortex can not rotate at all. Next, your energy channel that is connected with your dead useless vortex becomes cold and solid so that your energy channel is taken over by dirty energy bodies of others' and devils'. Your energy channel gets stuck by such as cold heavy oil, sludge, coal tar, cold clay, or solid snot. Your vortex, your energy channel can neither run fresh, useful energy of the universe and of the earth and of the spirit into your internal organ, nor evacuate bad energy and devils from your internal organ. The fire within your body goes out. The vortex of your body can neither rotate nor shoot out your immaterial fiber or third attention to an outside object so that you can neither judge an outside object nor change-control it.

At last, your internal organ that is connected with your dead, useless vortex and energy channel becomes cold and solid. Your internal organ gets stuck by such as cold heavy oil, sludge, coal tar, cold clay, or solid snot, and becomes almost dead or useless.

If your heart is stuck, your face will become dirty black red and horizontal line[about half an inch]will appear between your eyes. Red spots may happen to the back of your neck, too. If your liver is stuck, upper nose will become dirty blue or black blue. If your lung is stuck, your face will become dirty white. If your spleen is stuck, your face will become dirty yellow. If your kidney is stuck, your face will become dirty black and you will feel lazy about your legs. In all cases, your face will lose beautiful gloss.

Lump happens to your internal organ. There may exist disordered part of spine just at the back of your weak internal organ. Violent sports[soccer, rugby, and so on], intense exercise, Yoga, long meditation, or accident is apt to injure your spine. Stiff shoulder, not-rotating neck, and the peculiar feeling of your fingers[little pain, numb, impotent and so on]happen to you. Bad appetite, bad sleeping, bad bowel movement, and bad sex happen, too. Furthermore, your throat is apt to become weak or sore if you have divorced, been on bad terms with your wife or husband, or been much disappointed in love. It is because your throat is intimately connected with your sexual organ.

You are fearful of these warnings of your body. You go to 3-5 hospitals to check your body. But, nothing is problem with you in medical respect for 3-5 years. After that, cancer will happen to you, for example. As for heart disease or paralysis, it may happen to you in 1-6 months after these warnings of your body. A change for worse within your energy body, vortex, energy channel of your physical body and internal organ is, sticky-not glossy-fever-depressed-solid-cold-pass away. A change for better needs much wisdom and patience at least in 10 years. It is a big challenge. Trying a big challenge at your peril will surely make you much stronger, much more wise, patient and modest little by little than before. Maybe, one of many challenges at your peril is how to emerge from unfortunate vicious circle and beckon the spirit.

How to emerge from unfortunate vicious circle is as follows.

If we observe that we are coward, stingy, ironical, we need to strengthen our bodies and become healthier-Make our body stronger and more healthy with the help of some proper exercise such as constricting anus 100 times in succession and denting navel 100 times in succession everyday following the life style of long-lived British-A healthy appetite, good sleep, good bowel movement, good sex, give a good complexion and can make us look and feel younger than our age-Gradually the heart becomes stronger and more healthy-At times, we may experience that certain parts of the bodies feel hot, cold, painful or shivering-begin to rotate the vortexes of body-As the energy circulates from the abdomen to the head, it can happen that sometimes a small light (fire) twinkles within body which can erase stickiness and a sad or hateful personal history, so we can feel happier-This also makes us less coward, stingy, ironic in our action, speech and in the way we look at the world-It makes us practice abandon, largess, humor, also when speaking and in the way we look at the world-This enables us to occasionally begin to shoot out fairly well-developed immaterial fibers from the center of our abdomen and start to beckon the spirit-begin to succeed in concentrating on an outside object-supernatural power begin to happen to you-begin to follow the comfortable body-response obediently-We grow at least 10-20 years younger-Big explosions occur within head, chest, abdomen, or legs-Central energy-pipes in our bodies are cleaned up and begin to work again-At the abdomen big, pure, noble, strong, beautiful, dry, glossy light (fire) starts to develop-Inner silence is felt and it is possible to sleep without losing consciousness-It can happen that breath becomes very faint and sometimes stops naturally without dying-The third attention, silent knowledge, voice without voice, power of silence.

If what I have written reminds you, you will owe me much gratitude as a lifesaver when you can emerge from unfortunate vicious circle. In such a case, I feel pleased that you will save other people instead of returning a favor to me.

Furthermore, I think it is effective to cure or prevent depression and become happy-healthy-efficient that you (1)follow your body-response obediently(2)often check whether or not you eat in moderation, have good complexion, make friends with danger or death, have good self-importance, have dependable trust, have good repentance, burn the fire from within your body and clean up the central energy pipe of your body, walk in the right way, say thank you (3)stare at something with the middle of your eyebrows broadened and practice shooting out your immaterial fiber or third attention to an outside object from your body and control it for the purpose of succeeding in concentrating-The success of concentration can give more comfortable body-response, pleasure, healthy and efficiency to you(4)talk, see and act with abandon, largess and humor and can beckon the spirit (5)erase your bad stickiness and multiply various good feeling. I intend to explain them by turns.

# Part 4 Stare, shoot out immaterial fiber, succeed in concentrating, behave with abandon-largess-humor and beckon the spirit

**Stare, shoot out your immaterial fiber or third attention from your body, succeed in concentration and attain happy lucky feeling**

Goethe, the famous German Dramatist said "Enthusiasm can heal anything. If we do something seriously, we can heal ourselves. But, highbrow seldom does anything seriously". One of the ways to cure or prevent depression and become healthy-happy-efficient is to do something useful that can boil the head. You had better spend this minute as if it were your last.

I define a word of depression as not shooting out our immaterial fibers or third attention to an outside object from our bodies, being unable to judge it accurately, being unable to control it and being unable to concentrate on it so that we can not attain happy lucky feeling through the success of concentration and feel depressed. Concentration on something is the success of shooting out our immaterial fibers or third attention to something from our bodies so that we can judge it accurately, control it and can attain happy lucky feeling, inspiration, health and supernatural power.

Complaints (about opposite sex, son or daughter, parents, boss, health, money, work or post), dirty energy of others, devils and the trouble of spine give much dirty stickiness to our bodies and our aura so that they give bad complexion to us. Much dirty stickiness stops the rotation of our bodies' vortexes, makes the fire within our bodies go out and stop the movement of our immaterial fibers or of third attention so that we can not shoot out our immaterial fibers or third attention to an outside object, can not judge it accurately, can not control it. That is to say, we can not concentrate on an outside object and can not attain happy lucky feeling, inspiration, health or supernatural power through the success of concentration. In such a case, we feel dull and can have nothing that we are interested in or want to do with enthusiasm. If you feel dull and can have nothing that you are interested in or want to do with enthusiasm, I recommend that you keep on learning to do the Inca-style body-exercise called Tensegrity with enthusiasm for 4 hours everyday for a year.

Enthusiasm is shooting out our immaterial fibers or third attention to an outside object from our bodies, judging it accurately, controlling it, succeeding in concentrating on it and attaining happy lucky feeling, inspiration, health and supernatural power through the success of concentration.

Doing some proper body-exercise everyday such as constricting anus 100 times and denting navel 100 times following the life style of long-lived British can begin to erase the dirty stickiness of our bodies so that the vortexes of our bodies begin to rotate and the fire begins to burn from within our bodies. Then, we begin to feel energetic and have something that we are interested in or want to do with enthusiasm naturally. As a result, we can begin to have good complexion, make our immaterial fibers or third attention shoot out to an outside object from our bodies, judge it and control it easily. That is to say, we can succeed in concentrating on something or doing something with enthusiasm.

If you do not know the special pleasure of shooting out your immaterial fiber or third attention to an outside object from your body, of judging it accurately, of controlling it and of succeeding in concentrating on it, your world looks like a hell. The moment you shoot out your immaterial fiber or third attention to an outside object from your body and succeed in concentrating on it, you can begin to feel as if you fused with something and feel relieved and relaxed. You can begin to forget your pain, hate, depression or anxiety. You can begin to feel as if time stopped. You can begin to attain inspiration, pleasure, instinct, health and power through the success of concentration. Furthermore, you can begin to realize what you imagine, plan or think of because of the success of concentration.

Most of founders, big men, pioneers, masters and skilled craftsmen are not people with education and can do something with enthusiasm and in earnest after careful calculation as if they were crazy. Something is work, fight, challenge, adventure, love, study, research or hobby. They can turn to bay under a difficult condition as if they were crazy, too. In such a case, founders, big men, pioneers, masters and skilled craftsmen can shoot out their immaterial fibers or third attention to an outside object from their bodies and succeed in concentrating on it and attain happy lucky feeling, inspiration, pleasure, instinct, health and power through the success of concentration. They can succeed in concentrating on something within half an hour.

Furthermore, you will be able to get the secret of shooting out your immaterial fiber or third attention to your work, study or research from your body, of succeeding in concentrating on it and of attaining happy lucky feeling, inspiration, power naturally through the success of concentration if you keep on doing your work, study or research in earnest 8 hours everyday at least for 10 years. For example, in such a way, skilled craftsmen can gotten the secret of shooting out their immaterial fibers or third attention to their work from their bodies, of succeeding in concentrating on it and of attaining happy lucky feeling, inspiration, pleasure, instinct, health and power through the success of concentration.

A total of 10 million US people have entered the hospital because of depression. I think it is because Us people are apt to change jobs more easily and not do the same work earnestly and patiently at least for 10 years so that they can not get the secret of shooting out their immaterial fiber or third attention to their works from their bodies, of succeeding in concentrating on them and of attaining happy lucky feeling, inspiration, power naturally through the success of concentration. Furthermore, the divorces of themselves and of their parents and their big lost loves have given much complaint, sadness and hate to them so that they begin to have too much dirty stickiness of their bodies and of their auras. Then, the fires within their bodies go out because of too much their stickiness. The fires within their bodies can not burn out their dirty stickiness. As a result, the vortexes of their bodies and their immaterial fibers or third attention are confined to the too much dirty stickiness of their bodies and of their auras so that they can not move freely. Many US people can not shoot out their immaterial fibers or third attention to their work, fight, challenge, adventure, love, study, research or hobby from their bodies, can not succeed in concentrating on it and can not attain happy lucky feeling, inspiration, pleasure, instinct, health and power naturally through the success of concentration. Then, a total of 10 million US people must have entered the hospital because of depression.

In addition, executives and elite are apt to be such workaholics that they are too busy to sleep for more than 7 hours or too busy to do some proper body-exercise everyday. Little sleeping and not doing some proper body-exercise can weaken their bodies and hearts, and give much dirty stickiness to them, too. As a result, they can not shoot out their immaterial fibers or third attention to their works from their bodies because of their much dirty stickiness, can not judge their works accurately, can not control their works, can not succeed in concentrating on their works and can not attain happy lucky feeling, inspiration, pleasure, instinct, health and power naturally through the success of concentration. They will make bad decisions, fail in succession, become disgraced sooner or later. Then, they will suffer from depression, heart disease or cancer.

For the purpose of shooting out your immaterial fiber or third attention to something from your body, and of succeeding in concentrating on it easily, you had better get relaxed, broaden the middle of your eyebrows, walk enough, eat in moderation, forgive yourself or others, do good bowel movement, do some proper body-exercise, stop smoking, do not make unpleasant love, do not remember or meet unhappy-unhealthy-inefficient people, do not point the same aspect for long hours, have good complexion, sleep at least for 7 hours at night, stay at your power-spot and have good feelings such as those of light spring breeze, cunning, abandon, ruthless, largess, activity, sexiness, humor, clarity, sweet, fog, calmness, purification, kindness, bravery, patience, originality and detachment before you try to shoot out your immaterial fiber or third attention to something from your body and succeed in concentrating on it. If you do not do so before you try to shoot out your immaterial fiber or third attention to something from your body and concentrate on it, you seldom will be able to shoot out your immaterial fiber or third attention to something from your body, seldom will be able to concentrate on it, seldom will be able to attain happy lucky feeling, inspiration, power through the success of concentration.

Following your comfortable body-response, you had better select and have several things which you can shoot out your immaterial fiber or third attention to, concentrate on and attain happy lucky feeling, inspiration, power through the success of concentration easily. For you, such things are like a medicine, armor, castle, asylum, haven, radar, radiotelegraphy, missile, and weapon. In this respect, your life is the place where you have to learn the secret of shooting out your immaterial fiber or third attention to your work, fight, challenge, adventure, love, study, research or hobby from your body, of succeeding in concentrating on it and of attaining happy lucky feeling, inspiration, pleasure, instinct, health and power naturally through the success of concentration. If you can not learn such a secret, your life will look like a hell. Universities and graduate schools do not seem to teach such a secret. So, people with education are apt to suffer from depression more than uneducated people do.

To stare at the interspace between the leaves of a tree in a primeval forest or of a tree which has not been planted by human being-stare at the stone or rock which you like-stare at the star which you like for one hour everyday is one of the effective ways to practice shooting out your immaterial fiber or third attention to an outside object from your body, judging it accurately, controlling it so that you can succeed in concentrating on it and attain happy lucky feeling, inspiration, health and supernatural power through the success of concentration. The Second Ring of Power by Mr.Carlos Castaneda recommends it, too. It is much better that you stare with the middle of your eyebrows broadened for one hour everyday doing some proper body-exercise everyday such as constricting anus 100 times and denting navel 100 times.

Stare can bring up beautiful strong fire within your body so that this fire can burn or shut out the dirty stickiness that your complaint, dirty energies of other people and devils have given you. Your immaterial fiber or third attention that has been confined to the dirty stickiness of your body and of your aura can begin to move freely. As a result, you can shoot out your useful immaterial fiber or the third attention to an outside object from your body little by little, succeed in concentrating on it, attain happy lucky feeling and realize what you imagine or think of. You can lose undependable self-importance, undependable trust and self-pity. You can have dependable self-importance and dependable trust in yourself. Don Juan Matus, the Carlos Castaneda's teacher says about immaterial fiber or the third attention. He says "Without it, we are sediment or nothing".

Whenever you can realize what you imagine or think of, your body has not been taken over by the dirty stickiness that your complaint, dirty energy of other people or devil has given you. As a result, the fire within your abdomen has burned more beautifully and stronger. You do not feel stuck, irritated, depressed or gloomy. Then, good complexion, good bowel movement and soft shoulder have happened to you. In such case, you can shoot out your immaterial fiber or third attention to an outside object, judge-control it and realize what you imagine or think of more easily. That is to say, you succeed in concentrating on it, have dependable self-importance and self-confidence. The origin of your pleasure and of self-confidence is your strong beautiful fire within your body, your useful immaterial fiber or third attention and the success of concentration.

By and by, you can understand something that shoots out from the vortex on the surface of your body, and can catch on the object you stare at. Something is the immaterial fiber which shoot out from your body.

Furthermore, you will be able to see the aura of human being's, of animal's, and of tree's. At last, you will be able to see the aura of stone's, of rock's, of mountain's, river's, of sea's, of the ground's and of star's without using herbs.

After such a phenomenon, you may be able to feel that something beautiful, dry, glossy, sweet, kind, cool, active, nimble, fierce, peaceful, fluid and noble, will flow out of your body abundantly to the object you stare at or think about.

Such something is the third attention that can be compared to the inner spirit of yours or Phenix called God in Egypt. The third attention is much subtler, fainter than immaterial fiber which shoots out of your body. But, it is much stronger and nimbler than immaterial fiber. It has stronger attack-power and healing-power than immaterial fiber has. It can penetrate into or break through anything or any place immediately. It can travel to 2 billion light year distant-universe almost within a second. It is the origin of a seer, too. The origin of blue third attention is your healthy strong liver. The origin of red third attention is your healthy strong heart. The origin of yellow third attention is your healthy strong spleen. The origin of white third attention is your healthy strong lung. The origin of transparent third attention is healthy strong V-spot on the crest of the sternum at the base of your neck. The origin of black third attention is healthy strong kidney.

It is very difficult for us to confirm the existence of our subtle faint third attentions. The third attention can be compared to the smoke in a treasure-chest. Happy, healthy, or successful people have active useful third attention and use it in everyday life unconsciously. But, maybe, they will be at a loss about how to emerge from misfortune if they fall into misfortune and make their third attention dead and useless. They do not know how to make their third attention revive and work on for them again. Unhappy, unhealthy, or unfortunate people have dead useless third attention and have not made it work on for them unconsciously, so that they can not recognize the existence of the third attention at all. People who have neither active their useful third attention nor immaterial fibers can be compared to tigers without teeth in Africa or soldiers without guns on a battlefield.

Your active useful third attention can go out of your body and work on for you only while your breath is stopping automatically. Your breath is apt to stop automatically when you feel so happy that you want nothing and do not want to accomplish anything. If you want to confirm the existence of the third attention, you had better rent a house at your best power-spot place and keep on concentrating on your breath at your peril all day there for 3 weeks. You will experience hotness, coldness, shiver, pain, big explosion and big automatic whirl in your body. After 2 weeks you will be able to feel happy and stop your breath automatically. Then, your active useful third attention will begin to go out of your body and work on for you.

Indian Yoga book says "one who can stop one's breath automatically can attain or accomplish anything. You had better practice stopping your breath automatically several times everyday". If you are an

American, you can rent a house at your best power-spot place and challenge stopping your breath automatically at your peril when you are fired or change your job. I think you can clean up your life and appreciate my kindness. I have challenged it 5 times for 20 years.

Just before you can shoot out your immaterial fiber or the third attention from your body to the object which you stare at, concentrate on or think about, you have to stop your internal dialogue and enter into the peculiar inner silence or the peculiar happiness for a while. The feeling of stopping internal dialogue is such as putting a car into neutral or your being suspended .If you keep on staring at something everyday with the space between your eyebrows broadened, you will be able to stop your internal dialogue sooner or later, be able to shoot out your immaterial fiber or third attention to an outside object, be able to judge it and be able to control it. As a result, you will be able to succeed in concentrating on it, attain happy lucky feeling through the success of concentration and realize what you imagine or think of.

Stopping your internal dialogue, peculiar inner silence and peculiar happiness happen to you whenever you can stop your breath automatically. Then, you can shoot out your immaterial fiber or third attention to an object and judge-control it so that you can attain anything. Personal power is a lucky feeling or mood that can be brought about by stopping your internal dialogue and stopping your breath automatically. You can stop your internal dialogue and your breath automatically easily when good complexion, good appetite, good sleeping, good bowel movement, good sex, soft shoulder, rejuvenation, moderate eating, good waist and subtle breath happen to you.

After you can begin to see the aura of stone, you will be able to see something that is floating in the inner space, within the earth, or in the universe. Something is the spirit. It is blue, red, yellow, white, transparent, green, black, or orange. It is beautiful, dry, glossy, sweet, kind, cool, active, nimble, peaceful, fluid, noble, fierce, of abandon, of largess, and of humor.

At the beginning, your immaterial fiber may catch on many devils because your immaterial fiber is still dirty. Your immaterial fiber does not deserve to catch on the spirit. Furthermore, you may be tricked by devils and catch on many disguised devils because you are quite a stranger to another world.

You keep on staring at something and doing some proper body-exercise following the life style of long-lived British, or strengthening your energy by Chinese military arts everyday patiently. Then, you will be able to become much healthier, feel much happier than before, and your immaterial fiber will become beautiful, dry, glossy, sweet, kind, cool, active, nimble, peaceful, fluid, noble, fierce, of abandon, of largess, and of humor. As a result, your immaterial fiber will begin to catch on the spirit. Or, your third attention will begin to catch on the spirit.

The black spirit is often mistaken for devil. Dirty black one is one of devils. But, beautiful glossy one is the spirit that can give patience, originality and bravery to human being. It makes your bones strong, too. You will become arrogant if you absorb much energy of black spirit's through your kidney. You will be like a rotten female or rotten apple if you can absorb little energy of black spirit's. The yellow spirit can give you sweet. It makes your muscles healthy, beautiful, and strong. The yellow spirit is said to be the most important among the spirits. Such saying is not correct. If you stick to the yellow spirit and keep on absorbing only its energy too much, your abdomen will expand. You will feel irritated and often break wind. However nutritious and delicious food is, you will become bore, irritated, depressed, or unhealthy if you keep on eating it everyday for long time. That is the same. I hate the yellow spirit still now because I absorbed the energy of yellow spirit's too much 2 years ago.

The red spirit has ruthless joyful energy. The blue spirit has cunning energy. The black spirit has patient energy. The yellow spirit has sweet energy.

You can shoot out strong red immaterial fiber or third attention from healthy heart, catch on the red spirit, and absorb ruthless joyful energy from the red spirit. You can shoot out strong blue immaterial fiber or third attention from your healthy liver, catch on blue spirit and absorb cunning energy from the blue spirit. You can shoot out strong black immaterial fiber or third attention from your healthy kidney, catch on the black spirit, and absorb patient energy from the black spirit. You can shoot out strong yellow immaterial fiber or third attention from your healthy spleen, catch on the yellow spirit, and absorb sweet energy from the yellow spirit.

When your immaterial fiber or your third attention succeeds in contacting the spirit, the spirit will run something beautiful, dry, glossy, sweet, kind, cool, active, nimble, fluid, noble, fierce, of abandon, of largess, and of humor into you abundantly to strengthen, purify, heal or cure you. Such something is colorful or transparent. Such a phenomenon is the evidences to shoot out your immaterial or third attention to the spirit from your body and succeed in concentrating on it. Such a phenomenon has been said in China that you can succeed in rotating the vast universe. Don Juan Matus, the Carlos Castaneda's teacher says "Such a phenomenon is alignment" in the book with the title-The Fire From Within. Your energy's rotating automatically between your abdomen and head is said in China that you can succeed in rotating the small universe. It is the evidence that you can burn the fire from within your body.

You have to be aware whether you are stupid or wise. You have to be able to distinguish your inefficiency from your efficiency. When you are taken over by dirty stickiness that your complaints, dirty energy bodies of others and devils have given you, you can not rotate the vortexes of your bodies and feel stuck or depressed so that you can not shoot out the immaterial fiber or the third attention from your body and can not concentrate on. As a result, you can not realize what you imagine or plan and can not attain happy lucky feeling, inspiration, pleasure, instinct, health and power through the success of concentration. In such a case, you are stupid and inefficient. You look like a timid, stingy, gloomy man or woman. Then, you feel unhappy, sad, irritated, lonely, lazy, and impotent. A beautiful immaterial fire does not twinkle in your body so that your energy body is dirty, sticky, feverish, cold or solid. Bad complexion, bad appetite, bad bowel movement, poor or flabby abdomen, eating too much, bad sleeping, bad sex, stiff shoulder and rough breath happen to you.

When you are taken over neither by the dirty stickiness that your complaints, the dirty energy of others and devils can give you, a beautiful strong fire burns within your body and you have good complexion. In such a case, the vortexes of your body and your immaterial fiber or third attention have not been confined to the dirty stickiness of your body. The vortexes of your body can rotate smoothly and you can shoot out your immaterial fiber or the third attention to an outside object from your body easily. As a result, you can judge it accurately and control it so that you can succeed in concentrating on it and attain happy lucky feeling, inspiration, pleasure, instinct, health and power through the success of concentration. Then, you can realize what you imagine or plan so that you are self-confident, wise and efficient. You look like a man or woman of abandon, of largess, and of humor. A beautiful immaterial fire twinkles in your body so that your energy body is beautiful, dry, cool, or fluid. Good appetite, good bowel movement, moderate eating, soft and firm abdomen, good sleeping, good sex, flexibility of your body, and subtle breath happen to you naturally.

To be able to distinguish inefficiency from efficiency, you had better go into stupidity and inefficiency, and return to wisdom and efficiency intentionally many times. You had better be taken over by the dirty stickiness that your complaints, the dirty energy of others and devils can give you, and erase it intentionally many times. You had better catch on devil or the spirit by turns intentionally many times.

Furthermore, you had better remember your failures and successes in detail as possible at least 100 times, too.

Hey! According to the above-mentioned sentence, you had better test now whether or not your plan or idea (about money, work, post, hobby, opposite sex, friend, parents, son, daughter or health) can be realized sooner or later. In most cases, you can become aware that you have been confined to an undependable false plan or idea that is one of so-called hells on the earth. If you have an undependable false plan or idea, you can not burn the strong beautiful fire within your body, can not burn out the dirty stickiness of your body and of your aura, have bad complexion, feel dull, irritated, depressed, lonely, stuck or dreary. As a result, you can not shoot out your immaterial fiber or third attention to an object from your body, can not judge it accurately, can not control it, can not succeed in concentrating on it and ca not attain happy lucky feeling, inspiration, health or supernatural power through the success of concentration.

Needless to say, I have been confined to many such hells for long years. I have gone into stupidity-inefficiency and returned to wisdom-efficiency unconsciously many times. I have remembered my failures and successes in detail as many as possible, so I can barely have distinguished stupidity-inefficiency from wisdom-efficiency. As a result, I can have written about how to distinguish one from another to you. I feel I have paid many tuition fees for long years because of my stupidity and stubbornness.

After such a study, you have to be able to shoot out your strong immaterial fiber or the third attention from your body by all means when you have to be alert, wise, and efficient. Happy, healthy or successful people and skilled craftsmen can do so. You had better shoot out it to an outside object from your body, concentrate on it and attain happy lucky feeling, inspiration, pleasure, instinct, health and power through the success of concentration at least once everyday. If you do not do so everyday, your immaterial fiber or third attention will apt to become weak and almost dead, useless.

Gradually you will be aware that you can easily shoot out your strong immaterial fiber or the third attention to the outside object to which you have body-response such as (1)you begin to feel relieved and relaxed (2)begin to take a deep breath (3)stiff abdomen turns to be fluid and relaxed. Then, you will be aware that you can easily concentrate on the outside object to which your comfortable body-response happens and can easily control the outside object as you want. In such a case, you can easily attain happier luckier feeling through the success of concentration and realize what you imagine or think of.

Consulting our own interests or plausible reasons, most of us decide what to do or whether or not we make friends with someone or whether or not we marry someone without following body-response. Most of us just have to do anything. Most of us are not content to do. In such a case, we can neither shoot out our immaterial fibers or third attention to an outside object from our bodies nor concentrate on it so that we fail in realizing what we imagine or think of or plan. If we do so in succession, we begin to have much dirty stickiness of our bodies and make the fire within our bodies go out. As a result, our immaterial fibers or third attention begin to be confined to the dirty stickiness of our bodies and become almost dead and useless. Our immaterial fibers' or the third attention's being confined to our bodies for long time can weaken our bodies and hearts.

Then, most of us begin to have bad complexion, bad bowel movement, bad appetite, bad sleeping, bad sex and stiff shoulder. Happy lucky feeling (light spring breeze, cunning, ruthless, abandon, largesse, humor, joy, clarity, smooth, peace, sweet, calmness, purification, kindness, patience, bravery, originality, detachment, rushing headlong) runs away from our eyes, voices, behaviors so that we can not beckon the spirit, too. We become a toothless tiger. Most of us look like a slavery of money, food, post, fame or sex. In this respect, I have often failed because I have followed not my body-response but only my own interests or plausible reasons. So, you had better not make a decision only according to your own interests such as money, post, living, fame and sex. Following your comfortable body-response, you had better do as possible at your peril what you are content to do.

Now, you can understand "Shooting out your immaterial fiber or third attention to the object that you like from your body and succeeding in concentrating on it is the medicine for you. It can give you joy, pleasure and mercy, too. It is the way to cure or prevent depression, the way to become happy-healthy-efficient, the way to succeed in concentrating on something, the way to hunt power (happy lucky feeling) and inspiration. It is the same as the Buddhist precepts or the path of enlightenment or supernatural power or stopping your breath automatically or body-response or vanishing your pains and bad feeling or shutting out dirty shadow or vanishing devils or erasing your dirty stickiness or fusing with something or silent knowledge or seeing through or instinct or inner silence or realizing what you imagine easily or dependable trust", can't you?

It is the sentence of the book that was written in Chinese 2000 years ago by the prince of the big country just above Iran. He translated the teaching of Buddha into Chinese, explained it and wrote the book. It was very difficult for me to understand his book at the beginning 10 years ago. But, comfortable body-response happened to me. The core of my abdomen turned to be very hot and I felt as if all my body were burning while reading his book in Chinese. I had been staring at his book, shooting out my immaterial fiber or third attention to it and concentrating on it everyday since then as if I were solving a complicated puzzle. It took me 3 years to translate his book into Japanese, explain it and write the book with the title-How to concentrate on your breath and stop it automatically (in Japanese) 7 years ago.

I think most readers feel body-response such as feeling relieved or relaxed while reading my book even though most reader may not understand my book completely at the beginning. But, gradually most readers will be able to enjoy trying to understand my book further with the help of their immaterial fibers or third attention (body-response) as if most readers were solving a complicated puzzle. You can practice shooting your immaterial fiber or third attention and can bring up dependable trust while staring at and reading my book as many times as possible. Whenever you stare at my book, can shoot out your immaterial fiber or third attention to my book from your body, succeed in concentrating on my book and can understand some sentence of my book correctly and deeply, comfortable body-response happens to you. Then, your assemblage point (the core of your consciousness) breaks through the point of no self-pity and moves to the interior of the undoubted in your body. You can trust in "I can surely understand some sentence of this book "without a plausible reason. This is the way to read the letters of the ancient remains without dictionary, too. The future of your life looks like the letters of the ancient remains. So, you had better apply such a way at your peril to read the future of your life.

Furthermore, you had better make friends with danger or death at your peril. When you run a risk at your peril, you can burn the fire within your bogy, erase the dirty stickiness of your body easily, shoot out immaterial fiber or the third attention to an outside object from your body, succeed in concentrating on it and attain happy lucky feeling, inspiration, pleasure, instinct, health and power through the success of concentration. If you can not do so under a dangerous condition, you will be killed, seriously wounded or ruin.

Happy, healthy or successful people prefer running a risk. They are apt to like dangerous hobbies, too. They look like gentlemen and naughty boys. I think they seem to know that happy lucky feeling or pleasure has hidden behind danger. For those who do not know this secret, this world looks like a hell, too. The former US president, Geoge Bush enjoyed skydiving in summer in1999 in spite of his old age. I sometimes wonder if I buy a motorbike and mount it again although I am 59 years old. To the contrary, I think I will be ashamed if I am seriously wounded again or die of traffic accident. Mounting a motor-bike is very dangerous in Japan because of traffic jam. I was seriously wounded while mounting a motorbike about 30 years ago. 6 bones of my leg were broken and I had entered the hospital for 6 months.

Unhappy, unhealthy, unsuccessful people are like a rotten apple and hate running a risk at their perils. As a result, they can not burn the fire within their bodies, can not erase the dirty stickiness of their bodies easily, can not shoot out their immaterial fibers or the third attention to an outside object from their bodies, can not succeed in concentrating on it and can not attain happy lucky feeling, inspiration, pleasure, instinct, health and supernatural power through the success of concentration. One of the origins of rotten apples may be the shortage of beautiful glossy black energy and weak kidney.

To strengthen your immaterial fiber or your third attention, you had better strengthen your internal organ, physical body and energy body everyday, burn the fire within your body, erase your dirty stickiness, rotate the vortexes of your body, shoot out your immaterial fiber or third attention from your body, succeed in concentrate on something, attain happy lucky feeling through the success of concentration and catch on much stronger spirit as possible. The strength of the spirit is proportionate to the degree of the spirit's beauty, gloss, coolness, fluid, kindness, nimbleness, dignity, sweet, bloodthirstiness, nobleness, fierceness, abandon, largess, and humor.

We have to understand that we are giving a nuisance to a tree while we are staring at the interspace between a tree's leaves for 30 minutes-an hour. The tree feels painful, irritated or depressed because we are still dirty, sticky, feverish, cold, solid, numb, or rude. We can absorb less dirty, less sticky, less feverish, less cold, less solid, less numb, or less rude energy from a tree. A tree is a benefactor for us. So, we had better return the favor to a tree. At least, we had better not cut or break a tree mercilessly and unnecessarily from now on. If we can treat a tree as our friend as possible, it will turn to be our friend.

For the spirit or a tree, we are such as devils. We had better become more modest. For the earth, we are not more important or nobler than a tree. We only take and take from the earth, and soil the earth. We have not returned the favor to the earth.

While you are staring at an object, you had better touch or penetrate into softly and for a short time. You had better absorb the precious energy of object a little. Don't use and squeeze it until it has shriveled to nothing.

To practice shooting your immaterial fiber or third attention to an outside object from your body, concentrating on it and attaining happy lucky feeling, inspiration and power through the success of concentration, I recommend mainly that you had better stare at the interspace between the leaves of a tree in a primeval forest or of a tree which has not been planted by human being-stare at the stone or rock which you like-stare at the star which you like for one hour everyday. But, it is OK with you that you stare at anything that you like. In addition, it is OK with you that you practice shooting out your immaterial fiber or third attention to a smell, taste, sound, sense of touch or thought, concentrating on it and attaining happy lucky feeling, inspiration and power through the success of concentration. Some oversea Chinese visits and sniffs the smell of the site proposed for his factory. He does not believe in the plausible report which his junior partner visited and wrote about the site. Only when he shoots out his immaterial fiber or third attention to the smell of the site, concentrate on it and can sniff the good smell of the site, he will decide to make his factory there.

In such a case, I think that he shoots out his immaterial fiber or third attention to the smell of the site from around his nose.

When you practice shooting your immaterial fiber or third attention to an outside object from your body, concentrating on it and attaining happy lucky feeling through the success of concentration, you had better have 6 kinds of objects which can give you 6 different happy lucky feelings such as those of (1)light spring breeze, sprout of tree,

In this respect, we had better make friends with 6 different types of men or women.

A man of power has happy lucky feeling because he shoots out his immaterial fiber or third attention to anything, try to judge it accurately, try to control it not to be disgraced miserably so that he can succeed in concentrating on it and attain happy lucky feeling, inspiration and health through the success of concentration.

But, once he loses his power, he will become unhappy-unhealthy-inefficient soon and looks old. It is because he does not have to shoots out his immaterial fiber or third attention to an outside object, does not have to try to judge it accurately and does not try to control it not to be disgraced miserably so that he can not succeed in concentrating on it and can not attain happy lucky feeling, inspiration and health through the success of concentration. In addition, he will become too careless to concentrate on and can not attain happy lucky feeling, inspiration or health through the success of concentration because nobody watches all his behaviors in detail.

If you can not understand the strong beautiful fire within your body, the immaterial fiber, the third attention, the concentration or the happy lucky feeling triggered by the success of concentration at all, you had better ask some skilled craftsman or master about it. If you want to die not like a depressed animal in a safe zoo but like an animal in a dangerous Africa plain, you had better ask big men, founders, pioneers, enterprisers, gangsters or naughty boys whether or not a happy lucky feeling hides behind danger.

### Behave with abandon, largess and humor and can beckon the spirit

If we can act, talk or see with abandon, largess and humor, we can burn the fire from within our bodies, erase our dirty stickiness of our bodies which has stopped the rotation of our bodies' vortexes and shut our immaterial fibers or third attention. As a result, we can shoot out our immaterial fibers or third attention to an outside object, judge it accurately, control it so that we can succeed in concentrate on it, attain happy lucky feeling, inspiration, health and power and realize what we imagine or think of. Furthermore, we can burn the strong beautiful fire within our bodies. The spirit likes such a fire, approaches us immediately and gives happy feeling, inspiration, health and power to us, too.

Whenever we act like a coward, are stingy, of irony, talk like it, see the world in this way, then all energy bodies within and around our bodies become dirty, dark, sticky or solid, causing a fever of depression, or coldness. This attracts devils which torture us. On the other hand however, whenever we do the acts of abandon, largess, humor, speak and look at the world in this way, some part of our energy bodies starts to flash, twinkle, or shine beautifully so that we can begin to feel a peculiar happy feeling and cure depression, too. The spirit find such beautiful fires in our energy bodies immediately, approach us at full speed, and help us, because the spirit likes beautiful immaterial fires in our energy bodies very much.

I think that it is the same in the relationship between men and women. Whenever men act out of abandon, largess, humor, talk in this way and looks though such eyes, men twinkle beautiful immaterial fires in their energy bodies. Women then can feel something special or happy about these men and approach them although most of women can not see beautiful immaterial fires of these men. Maybe, many women would like to be loved by these men quietly.

I think, beautiful immaterial fire in your energy body triggered by the acts of abandon, of largess, of humor, by talking in such voices, by seeing through such eyes is a noble offering of delicious scattered food or good pheromone to beckon the spirits, opposite sex, furthermore, health, rejuvenation, longevity, happiness, joy, friends, money, high position, and so on. Yoga book also says "If you recite a short sentence more than one or two million times and burn a beautiful strong fire within your body, you will be loved by many women or female angels (one of the spirits)".

How about you now?could it be that you are not satisfied with your life? Don't hold grudge against others. One could say that you feel this way because you may have rather offered rotten fruits, meats or even your excrement. Make sure you offer noble, delicious offerings carefully to people, your body, your heart and the spirits to be able to say "I am satisfied ". Be careful not to become proud. You had better keep on offering a noble delicious offering carefully to people, your body, your heart and the spirit.

For most of us, practicing abandon, largess, humor, talking in such a manner and seeing through such eyes become very difficult when our complaints (about opposite sex, son or daughter, parents, boss, money, work or post), the dirty energy of others and devils have given much dirty stickiness to us. In such a case, both the rotation of our bodies' vortexes has been stopped by our dirty stickiness and the fire within our bodies has been gone out by it. Our internal organs and our bodies are weak and unhealthy. Our immaterial fibers or third attentions have been confined to the dirty stickiness of our bodies and can not shot out to an outside object from our bodies, so that we can not judge it accurately, can not control it, can not concentrate on it and can not attain happy lucky feeling, inspiration or supernatural power through the success of concentration. Then, we can not realize what we imagine or think of. As a result, most of us have the tendency towards cowardice, stinginess, irony, also speak in such a way, and see through such eyes, no matter how persistently we want to avoid it. As a result of such acting, talking, and seeing, most of us can not attract the spirit when we need its help of the spirit the most.

Consequently, most of us will tend to be of more complaint, grudge, pain, illness, worry or grieve, of less abandon, less largess and less humor. And what's more we may start believing that there is no spirit or God. This is vicious circle.

Those who have been attracting their spirits, will not be able to beckon them once they get into this vicious circle. Their spirits will hate them and fly away from them. However once they realize that and emerge from it, they will be able to beckon their spirits again.

To act, talk or see with abandon, largess and humor, we had better constrict anus 100 times in succession and dent navel 100 times succession everyday at first following the life style of long-lived British so that we can begin to erase the dirty stickiness of our bodies, rotate the vortexes of our bodies and burn strong beautiful fire within our bodies, have good complexion and become happy and healthy. When we can begin to erase the dirty stickiness of our bodies, rotate the vortexes of our bodies and burn strong beautiful fire within our bodies, have good complexion and become happy and healthy, we want to act, talk and see with abandon, largess and humor naturally. Since then, we have to practice acting, talking or seeing with abandon, largess and humor in your ordinary world everyday to beckon the spirit. When the spirit touch you, you can burn the fire within your body more beautifully and strongly, can shoot out your immaterial fiber or third attention from your body and concentrate on something more easily. The spirit can give you much more happiness, inspiration, health, and supernatural power. You can realize what you imagine or think of with the help of the spirit.

These good examples are Mr.Rodney. H. Browne (in Florida, U.S.A, from South Africa), Mr.Carlos Annacondia (Argentine), Mr. Morris Cerullo (Jew), Mr. Steve Ryder (Australian). They are preachers or ministers.

Four preachers can knock down, fall down, or faint their audiences for 30 seconds up to one hour without using their arms or feet. Four preachers can cure the diseases, deformities in people while they fainted, were knocked or fell down during their group sessions.

They can also change the characters of their audiences and give much joy to them. They can improve the lives of their audiences, for example in regard to financial provision. Furthermore, Mr.Carlos Annacondia and Mr. Steve Ryder said in Japan that they could revive dead persons. They have visited Japan and I have attended their event since 3 years ago. I was able to see their mysterious, powerful, and kind ability before my eyes in Japan.

They have said to their audiences that they can cure the diseases of their audiences and change the lives of their audiences only when the spirit (they have often called it God)visits them and works on their audiences through them.

To beckon the spirit, entice it, become familiar with it and express it with their acts, they act out of abandon, largess, and humor. They are bringing out the best of themselves and offer it to the spirit before their audiences begin to fall and get knocked down, or faint. I think that they are warriors, too, according to the book, the Power of Silence by Mr.Carlos Castaneda, although they are preachers or ministers. It is because they can beckon the spirit. Furthermore, it is because they can shoot out their immaterial fibers to an object (their audiences) from their abdomen and judge-control it.

The spirit is abstract, intent, and God because the spirit looks like red, white, blue, transparent or yellow fog or gas or light that has intent, emotion and silent knowledge. The spirit can immediately penetrate into anybody, anything or any place, and travel into the interior of the universe at super high speed faster than that of a light. The spirit is floating in the air, inside the earth and in the universe. It is abstract, empty, but it can immediately turn into any definite immaterial body if it wants.

I think the color of the spirit is not only of dark gold dust, but also of different colored dusts. The spirits ( knowledge )are different in character, ability, color, smell, contact-feeling, sound, speed and temperature one after another.

The spirit becomes much stronger and nimbler in proportion to the degree of the spirit's dryness, nobleness, gloss, kindness, weakness, clearness, and sweet. There are many strong and nimble spirits who seem to be weak on first sight. That is the same as among human beings. Strong and agile men often seem to be weak on first sight.

The spirit of Mr. Morris Cerullo, and the spirits of former US presidents of Geoge Bush and Reagan, US vice-president Albert Gore, seem to be weak, sweet and kind on first sight, but they are really very strong.

The color of Mr. Morris' spirit is blue, transparent, and white. He often said "I am a Jew and an orphan. My parents died when I was 2 years old. I was raised in an orphanage". He said in June in 1998 in Japan" I preached 30 thousand Haitians and fought against 300 Haitian witches who came to my ministerial meeting and tried to kill me".

The color of Mr. Reagan's spirit is white blue. Mr. Reagan's spirit seems to be weak and sweet, but really incredibly enormous. His spirit can disarm anybody without orders or threat, and can use anybody freely without orders. Anybody is apt to follow his spirit voluntarily. Many people wondered why this third rate actor was able to elected as the president of U.S.A. Many people thought" I seem to have better head than that of Mr. Reagan's". I think that his incredible, enormous spirit loved Mr.Reagan and led to his being elected.

Similarly, the spirits of Mr.Geoge Bush, of Mr. Albert Gore are weak and sweet on first sight, but really strong and immense. The spirit of Mr. Bush is of red-orange color, has a secret weapon like a sharp dagger side-thrown by hand, and can enlarge to the same width of the state of California about 2 thousand km high. I can feel Mr. Bush has become more powerful, excellent, healthier and happier than during the presidency of U.S.A. He would become much better president than before. I can see that his son has begun to climb a beautiful tense rope upward slowly which the universe hangs since summer in 1999. The beautiful strong spirit has begun to touch his son and make his son flash since spring in 1999.

The spirit of Mr. Gore is of noble transparent color and has the mood of noble silent weak old woman, but has a secret weapon like a sharp needle which stabs the medulla oblongata of enemies' without their noticing it, and has a better head than computer. I think that if Mr.Gore becomes the president of U.S.A, the peculiar silence, peace, cool, sharpness, and sweet of his spirit will govern our earth.

Although these 3 big men in the political world of U.S.A have not practiced special training for warriors, and shamans, I think they are also warriors and modern shamans because they have been much loved by their spirits. I am sure they have been of so much abandon, of so much largess, of so much humor that they have been much loved by their spirits. I think many women must have liked them, too.

Mr.Rodney. H. Browne succeeded in beckoning the spirit in 1979 in South Africa for the first time. He had been thirsting and hungering for the spirit, and been praying and crying" Give me your power?""Fire? burn?be filled". Then, the spirit with the character of fire suddenly descended into him, so that the living water began to overflow from the bottom of his abdomen.

Mr.Rodney. H. Browne began to laugh, cry and talk in unknown voices, and had been drunken by the spirit of fire for 3 days. He felt as if he might die. He has big white energy pipe on his back that is half a foot in diameter and 5 feet in length. He has the black red spirit who is joyful, courageous, strong, immense, sweet, of abandon, of largess, and of humor. His spirit is such as a super tidal wave or a super wing-bird. I think he has much hidden ability to become a good psychic astronaut if he wants. His spirit can overflow Japan in 2 seconds, or make a vertical take-off and landing that could be compared to an aircraft.

But, I wonder why Mr.Rodney. H. Browne does not reduce his body weight. He is too fat, which gives his voice a painful tone, and his aura and his energy body are not very dry but a little sticky (human form called by Mr. Carlos Castaneda). I believe that his being obese must be the cause of diabetes, heart disease or cerebral hemorrhage, sooner or later. I wonder why his spirit(he calls it God)has not advised him to lose much of his weight because his spirit has been advising him to succeed in the U.S.A in only 12 years.

He said that he emigrated to U.S.A with only about 300 dollars in 1987, could not afford to buy a car for 7 months after his emigration. He is now 39 years old. By the grace of his spirit' good advises, he has succeeded in U.S.A to held his big mission-meeting at Madison square garden in New York from July 7 to August 13 in 1999.

Personal power is a lucky or happy feeling. I think Mr.Rodney. H. Browne will feel a feeling of being much luckier or happier if he succeeds in reducing his body weight. Mr.Rodney. H. Browne will become much more powerful and give much more joy to more people, and save more people if he succeeds in reducing his body weight. I expect he will be able to do so.

Mr. Carlos Annacondia ran a screw plant in Argentine. He had about 80 employees. He had been thirsty and hungry for the spirit and prayed for the spirit. Then, the spirit descended into him. Following the voice of his spirit, he gave up his business and became a preacher. This was during Falcon Island War. He said that he knew only one story of the Scriptures at that time, so he started to preach at slums to exaggerate one story of the Scriptures to gain time. He often said "The way to open the gate of heaven(to beckon the spirit)is to forgive yourself and others". He said "One day, a young crippled women was crying {I forgive my father} in succession loudly at his meeting, then threw down a pair of her crutches, and could begin to walk without them".

When Mr. Carlos Annacondia visited Japan in September in 1998. I saw his spirit is transparent and green where a noble female angel and a plump male live. This noble female angel dislikes the plump male whose color is black and yellow. I said to this plump male "Don't worry Mr. Annacondia". Many people have stopped smoking drug where Mr.Carlos Annacondia has come and preached, so many gangs have tried to assassin him with guns or rifles. But, the gangs have failed to kill him because Mr. Carlos Annacondia made them faint during his session without using his arms or feet while they held guns and riffles. This is the proof that he has a highly developed and strong immaterial fiber that shot out to gangs from his abdomen and fainted gangs.

Highly developed and strong immaterial fiber is a qualification of a warrior, or shaman. Furthermore, A Separate Reality says that "(inner) intent(a bunch of well-developed strong immaterial fibers) is what can make a man succeed when his thought tells him that he is defeated.(Inner)intent is what makes him invulnerable. The biggest purpose of a warrior or shaman is to revive practically dead, useless(inner)intent which dose not respond voluntarily. An average man has practically dead, useless(inner)intent which dose not respond voluntarily".

Don. Juan. Matus, Yaqui Indian, the teacher of Mr.Carlos Castaneda said "We are sediment or nobody without(inner)intent(highly developed strong immaterial fibers)". They should be like those of Mr. Carlos Annacondia to shoot out to gangs from the center of his abdomen and fainted gangs whenever they tried to assassin Mr. Carlos Annacondia in Argentine.

Not only Mr. Carlos Annacondia but also Mr. Morris Cerullo, Mr.Rodney. H. Browne, Mr. Steve Ryder have plenty of their highly developed strong immaterial fibers which shoot out to their audiences from the centers of their abdomens. This makes their audiences knock down or fall down and faints them.

When Mr. Carlos Annacondia preached in September in 1998 in Japan, he seemed to be tired at first. But, he turned to be much powerful when he began to look up constantly and a barrel of nectar at the top of his head suddenly flowed down his body. He has had the most nectar among the people whom I have seen. His nectar is cool, pure, noble, and fragrant, which can cure disease, give much peace. The book, Journey to Ixtlan by Mr.Carlos Castaneda says about the same kind of nectar that flowed down from the top of Mr.Carlos Castaneda's head at his best power-spot place in Mexico. Such nectar can erase a man's personal history (bad self-importance, hate, sadness and self-pity) and a man's dirty stickiness(human form), and lead a man into inner silence that can beckon the spirit.

Mr. Steve Ryder(born in 1937)said "I was a bank robber, and sentenced to be in prison for 20 years in Australia". When he was on parole, he heard the preach of the Billy Graham Crusade that" One is saved who believes in God". He thought that I was a parolee, sentenced to be in prison for 20 years, and unhappy. He thought he would be able to believe in God if God gave him the same power as that of Christ's. He was wondering what gift would be given to him by God without eating food for 3 days. At one point, he wanted to enter into a basement room of a certain hospital in Australia. He entered into this room and the spirit, like white gas engulfed him. While he was going out this room and walking along the corridor of the hospital, the nurses he encountered fainted.

Mr. Steve Ryder said to his audiences in Japan "I was arrested for armed robbery, sentenced to be in prison for 20 years, and lives vigorously now. Please, have courage in your heart if you are of pain, illness, worry, or grieve in your life". His message had big punch, much persuasiveness and strong impression.

I recommend my readers to attend a meeting which Mr.Rodney. H. Browne (his church, River at Tampa-Bay in Florida in U, S, A), Mr. Carlos Annacondia, Mr.Morris Cerullo or Mr.Steve Ryder (Reach out for Christ international ministries) will hold. Watch their gestures, hear their voices and see their eyes, so that you can understand why they can beckon the spirits. Their gestures are acts of abandon, of largess, of humor. The mood of their voices and eyes are full of abandon, of largess, of humor. Imitate their acts and the moods of their voices, of their eyes if you have not yet been loved by the spirit and you thirst for being loved by the spirit. Buy their tapes and listen to their voices at least 100 times, too.

Also observe the actions, voices and eyes of former US president. Geoge Bush or vice-president of U.S.A. Albert Gore who have the moods of abandon, largess, humor, and not forget their moods. Buy the tapes of speeches by former US president Reagan which were recorded in his greatest glory, and listen 100 times.

This will enable you to distinguish the voice which can beckon the spirit, from the voice which can not beckon the spirit, sooner or later. I think their spirits will begin to appear in front of you, begin to love you, and begin to give you some or small part of the same power.

After this, detect the voices of the nature, of the inner-earth, of the universe which can give you happiness and power, and hear their voices as many times as possible. You will be healed to remember the moods of these voices if you are tired or depressed. That is to say, you can beckon the spirit floating in the nature, the inner-earth or the universe. The scriptures say that sheep can detect the voices of a shepherd and only follow them.

At present, most pastors seem to be unable to beckon the spirit and unable to have supernatural power. Most pastors pray, sing, read the Scriptures and worry about management (money?). They are apt to go anywhere by car, eat too much, apt not to walk enough and apt not to do some proper body-exercise. They have wives and do not seem to save sex energy. In such a case, it is very difficult that they can burn the beautiful strong fires within their body, erase the dirty stickiness of their bodies, rotate the vortexes of their bodies, shoot out their imma- terial fibers or third attention to an outside object from their bodies, concentrate on it, attain happy lucky feeling, inspiration and power through the success of concentration, and realize what they imagine or think of. As a result, most pastors act, talk or see with less abandon, less largess and less humor so that the spirit can not find beautiful strong fires within their bodies, hate them and does not help them.

The reason why 4 pastors, Mr.Rodney. H. Browne(in Florida, U.S.A, from South Africa), Mr.Carlos Annacondia(Argentine), Mr. Morris

Cerullo(Jew), Mr. Steve Ryder(Australian) can burn the fire within their bodies and beckon the spirit is that their lives have been full of abandon, largess and humor. Especially, they are apt to talk or preach from the bottom of abdomen with abandon, largess and humor everyday. If we recite a short sentence from the bottom of abdomen with abandon, largess and humor for 4 hours everyday at least for 3 years, we can suddenly burn the beautiful strong fires within their bodies and beckon the spirit. So, they can burn the beautiful strong fires within their bodies and beckon the spirit, too. Furthermore, they have much ability to succeed in concentrating on something. They have thirsted for the spirit and succeeded in concentrating on the spirit owing to their much ability to succeed in concentrating on something.

If you can not understand that the spirit can give us happy lucky feeling, inspiration, health and supernatural power at all, you had better read the Scriptures carefully many times. The Scriptures is the book which has introduced many examples that the spirits approached, invaded into Jewish people and helped them. Furthermore, you had better ask founders, big men, pioneers, enterprisers or masters about the spirit because they are apt to act, talk or see with abandon, largess and humor so that they can burn the strong beautiful fires within their bodies which can beckon the spirit. Most of us can not understand the spirit at all and regard the people who talk about the spirit as insane. So, founders, big men, pioneers, enterprisers and masters have kept the spirit in secret and received happy lucky feeling, inspiration health and supernatural power from the spirit in secret.

When I did 3-week fasting at a center of fasting one and half an years ago, I met an old female master at stringed instrument called koto. She was 85 years old and entered a center of fasting to refresh herself. She played a koto in front of the late Japanese emperor, Hirohito. She had practiced playing koto for 8-10 hours everyday for 50-60 years since the age of 15.

cunning (2)ruthless, abandon, joy, self-confidence, sexiness (3)transparen (4)sweet (5)kindness, insanity and genius, purification, moderate sadness (6)detachment, patience, bravery, fight, originality, rushing headlong the moment you can succeed in concentrating on.

The happy lucky feeling of (1) can strengthen liver. But, your liver weakens if you only attain the too much happy lucky feeling of (1). The happy lucky feeling of (2) can strengthen your heart. But, your heart weakens if you only attain the too much happy lucky feeling of (2). The happy lucky feeling of (3) can strengthen your V-spot of your throat. But, your V-spot weakens if you only attain the too much happy lucky feeling of (3). The happy lucky feeling of (4) can strengthen your spleen. But, your spleen weakens if you only attain the too much good feeling of (4). The happy lucky feeling of (5) can strengthen your lung. But, your lung weakens if you only attain the too much happy lucky feeling of (5). The happy lucky feeling of (6) can strengthen your kidney. But, your kidney weakens if you only attain the too much happy lucky feeling of (6).

Some famous saint who preached about love always watched the violent scenes of TV. The people who knew him could not understand his inconsistent behavior. If he had behaved with love all day, he would have attain the too much happy lucky feeling of sweet so that his spleen would have weakened because of too much of sweet. So, he prevented his spleen from weakening instinctively owing to shooting his immaterial or third attention to the violent scenes of TV, concentrating on them and attaining the happy lucky feeling of bravery and of rushing headlong. To the contrary, gangsters and heroes are apt to love females, their families and pets very much. They often have such a strange inclination that they never kill a mosquito, insect or fry. If they behaved with bravery, fight and rushing headlong all day, their kidneys would weaken. The sweeter you are, the crueler you have to become. The crueler you are, the sweeter you have to become.

She said to me "I can not play my koto well unless I can shoot out my energy to the sound of my koto and fuse with the sound of my koto. Only when I can shoot out my energy to the sound of my koto and fuse with it, I feel as if I fused with something mysterious and play my koto well. When I have to sing a song while playing a koto, I always sing a song from the bottom of my abdomen. I often can foresee many thing accurately". Her energy that she shoots out to the sound of her koto is her immaterial fiber or third attention. Her fusing with the sound of her koto is the success of concentrating on the sound of her koto. Her feeling as if she fused with something mysterious and playing her koto well is her beckoning the spirit and fusing with the spirit. Her foreseeing many things accurately is her shooting out her immaterial fiber or third attention to an outside object from her body and judging it accurately. She has prayed to sunrise every morning for many years. While praying, she always sees a beautiful light or beautiful image in the sky although cloud or rain hides sunrise. A beautiful light or beautiful image in the sky is one of the spirits.

Furthermore, it is one of the effective ways to burn the beautiful strong fire within your body, erase the dirty stickiness of your body, rotate the vortexes of your body, shoot out your immaterial fiber or third attention to an outside object, judge it accurately, control it, succeed in concentrating on it, attain happy lucky feeling, inspiration and supernatural power through the success of concentration and realize what you imagine or think of that you keep on singing a song, preaching, praying or reciting a short sentence from the bottom of your abdomen for 4 hours everyday at least for 3 years.

Needless to say, 4 above-mentioned pastors have kept on singing a song, preaching, praying or reciting a short sentence from the bottom of their abdomens for long hours everyday for many years. They also sing a song, preach, pray or recite a short sentence with abandon, largess, humor, enthusiasm and earnest. It is one of the reasons why they can burn the beautiful strong fire within their bodies, shoot out their immaterial fibers or third attention to their audiences, beckon the spirit, faint them without using their arms or feet and cure many diseases. An Argentine pastor, Carlos Annacondia can faint many gangsters to try to assassin him without using his arms or feet and could revive the dead. He can have begun to do so since 3 years later after he began to preach from the bottom of his abdomen with abandon, largess, humor, enthusiasm and earnest. I hear some female Italian singer can break a glass cup with her song. I guess she has kept on singing a song from the bottom of her abdomen with abandon, largess and humor for long hours every day for long years and burned a beautiful strong fire within her abdomen. But, regrettably, most pastors and most of us apt to utter voices not from the bottom of abdomen but from mouth or chest everyday for many years. In addition, most pastors and most of us seem to utter voices with cowardice, stinginess, cynicism and lethargy for many years. That is the way it goes.

Yoga book says "if you recite a short sentence more than one million or 2 millions times, you will begin to have supernatural power and be love by young women and angels. The boss devil who has control your region will become your junior partner at last". My dear friend, a surgeon who has run the surgery hospital has kept on reciting a short sentence from the bottom of his abdomen for 2 hours in the morning and for 2 hours at night everyday for 8 years. He can have begun to faint people without using his arms or feet and cured cancer without operation since 5 years ago. In addition, you had better recite a short sentence with abandon, largess and humor, enthusiasm and earnest if you try to recite it from the bottom of your abdomen. Then, you can easily burn the beautiful strong fire within your body, erase the dirty stickiness of your body, rotate the vortexes of your body, shoot out your immaterial fiber or third attention to an outside object, judge it accurately, control it, succeed in concentrating on it, attain happy lucky feeling, inspiration and supernatural power through the success of concentration, realize what you imagine or think of and beckon the spirit.

# Part 5 Erase your bad stickiness and multiply various good feeling

## Erase your bad stickiness

Your third attention that hides within your body is like a smoke in a treasure-chest. How to recognize and handle it for you. Erasing stickiness make it appear from your body.

The earth is coiled round by something such as immaterial melted plastic. Inner space is like a band of immaterial melted plastic. Such something flows from the south to the north on the surface of the earth like a large river about at speed of a foot per second.

When sun beam begins to hit the margin of the band just before sun-rise, the band sings a song like thousands of birds. Sunbeam begins to invade into the band and makes the smell of something burning emit in the band. Some part of the sunbeam can not break though the band, and is divided on the margin of the band. It engulfs the margin of the band. The band of the earth is very sticky. The band of the earth seems to prevent the earth from bursting. This band is equal to the sticky first attention of human being's body.

If your immaterial fiber or third attention wants to venture out to the rustling and dry universe, it has to be able to break through such sticky inner space. If your immaterial fiber or third attention is sticky, it can not break through sticky inner space. Your sticky immaterial fiber or third attention is caught in the sticky inner space. Your complains, dirty energy bodies of others and devils can have given much dirty stickiness to your immaterial fiber or third attention. If your immaterial fiber or third attention is rustling and dry, it can break through sticky inner space.

Tree, stone and star can give you rustle and dryness. So, to erase your dirty stickiness, you had better stare at tree, stone, or star with your eyebrows broadened everyday for 30 minutes-an hour for 10 years doing some proper body exercise such as constricting anus 100 times and denting navel 100 times everyday following the life style of long-lived British. Furthermore, to erase your dirty stickiness, you had better do 3-week fasting, have good complexion, turn to bay, follow your comfortable body-response, have dependable good self-importance and dependable trust, eat in moderation, repent deeply, stay at your power-spot, succeed in concentrating on something, make friends with danger or death, act, talk and see with abandon, largess and humor, recite a short sentence from the bottom of abdomen with abandon, largess and humor, and concentrate only on your inhalation and exhalation all day for 3 weeks or concentrate only on your inhalation and exhalation everyday as possible, too. In addition, to erase your stickiness, Yoga book recommends (1)swallow down 3,5 m long cloth slowly and draw it under the supervision of the teacher (2)inject water into anus and move the muscle of abdomen (3)insert a piece of string into nose and draw it from mouth under the supervision of the teacher (4)stare at a small object until you shed tears (5)turn the muscle of abdomen (6)breathe fast like bellows.

If you practice the above mentioned contents, you will be able to begin to burn the beautiful strong fire within your body, burn out your much dirty stickiness of your body and of your aura, release your immaterial fiber or the third attention from your dirty stickiness. As a result, you can shoot out your immaterial fiber or the third attention from your body, catch on tree, stone, or star through it, and absorb the rustling and dry energy from tree, stone, or star. Your immaterial fiber or your third attention will become less sticky and more rustling and drier. Furthermore, You can shoot out your immaterial fiber or third attention to an outside object from your body, concentrate on it and attain happy lucky feeling inspiration, health and supernatural power through the success of concentration after you practice the above mentioned contents, can begin to burn the beautiful strong fire within your body, burn out your much dirty stickiness of your body and of your aura and release your immaterial fiber or the third attention from your dirty stickiness.

After you can shoot out rustling and dry immaterial fiber or third attention from your physical body, you will be able to let it break through the sticky inner space and fly into the far distant rustling and dry universe immediately.

Furthermore, you can shut out dirty energy bodies of others and devils if you begin to have more rustling or dry immaterial fiber or third attention, aura and body. Dirty energy bodies of other' and devils can neither live in rustling and dry immaterial fiber or third attention, aura and body nor stick to rustling and dry ones. They hate rustling and dry immaterial fiber or third attention, aura and body and like sticky ones. So, they live in or stick to sticky immaterial fiber or third attention, aura and body of human being, and sticky inner space.

The spirit hates sticky immaterial fiber or third attention, aura and body of human being, and sticky inner space. It likes rustling and dry immaterial fiber or third attention, aura and body of human being, rustling, dry universe and inner earth. A power-spot on the earth has a hole and is connected with the rustling, dry universe by the long energy cylinder. So, power-spot is not sticky. The spirit is floating at a power spot on the earth, too.

Besides dirty energy bodies of others and devils, complaint has given you much dirty stickiness. There are many kinds of complaints. I think the second or third biggest complaint is the bad relationship with opposite sex, or with son or daughter. Disease is the first biggest complaint. I think the bad relationship with parents is the fourth biggest complaint. The fifth biggest one is the complaint about work, money and post.

I think there exists fair impartiality about complaints. Most of us have a certain complaint more or less. We can have neither all good fortunes nor all misfortunes. Those who have been proud of their good fortunes are apt to ruin in 3-5 years, at the latest in 10 years.

I think the bad relationship with an opposite sex is the second biggest obstacle to cure or prevent depression and become healthy or efficient.

If one has divorced or lost a big love, one will be given much stickiness by it. One will be given much stickiness by the bad relationship with a spouse and the death of a spouse, too. Stickiness will make one's vortexes on the surface of one's body, the energy channels of one's internal organ, internal organ and the central energy pipe of one's body get stuck.

So, beautiful immaterial fire will go out and not be able to twinkle in one's body. Bad complexion, bad appetite, bad bowl movement, bad sleeping, bad sex, stiff shoulder will happen. Intimately throat is connected with sex organ through energy channel. So, one's throat is apt to become sore or a malign tumor because of the bad relationship with your opposite sex such as divorce, big lost love or the death of spouse. One's voice is apt to become bad. One will feel unhappy, lonely, depressed, irritated. One's immaterial fiber of one's body will become almost dead and useless. One can not shoot out one's immaterial fiber from one's body, so that one can not catch on the spirit that can give human being happiness-health-ability. Needless to say, one can not shoot out the third attention from one's body. Cancer is apt to happen, sooner or later.

I think Mr. Carlos Castaneda could not have become the successor to don Juan Matus, the teacher of Mr. Carlos Castaneda because he parted from the woman who had his child. Although he was taught how to get rid of his stickiness by don Juan Matus, he seemed not be able to have gotten rid of his stickiness almost completely. The bad relationship with the opposite sex seemed to have given him much stickiness, the fever of depression, coldness, and numbness.

I think the big origin of Napoleon's downfall was his divorce from his wife whom he loved. His wife could not have his baby, so he divorced although he loved her. She seemed to be a flirt, too. The sadness gave him considerable stickiness and the fever of depression, and become weak, so his abdomen often itched. The itch made his immaterial fiber or his third attention weak and undependable. With weak and undependable one, he nearly became like a teethless tiger. I imagined about him staring at his coffin in Paris.

If we are intimate with opposite sex, we can not save our sex energy. If we are not full of sex energy, we will lose the same noble fierceness as that of a young hawk so that our immaterial fibers or third attention can not break through the sticky inner space. If we can shoot out the immaterial fiber or the third attention from our bodies, it will be apt not to go straight but to bend and fall because of sex energy's lack. It can not reach an object. A moderate relationship with a spouse is apt to give subtle stickiness. It is very difficult for us to be conscious of subtle stickiness and to get rid of it. It can be compared to alloy in fuel.

Although some American woman has been doing Inca-style body exercise called Tensegrity earnestly for long years as to teach it to others, she had had much sad stickiness in her womb until 2 years ago. When I met her 2 years ago, I was much surprised to find that her womb was full of sad stickiness. As soon as I made her get rid of it, the strong noble white immaterial fiber shot out from her body to the sky.

Like Napoleon, my father was beaten not by a gun or sword but by the bad relationship with opposite sexes. My father was a lieutenant of Japan army and very brave in a battlefield. But, after World War 2, he got stuck by much stickiness because of the bad relationship with my mother.

My father's first wife died in childbirth. My father loved his first wife very much. My mother is a second wife of my father. After World War 2, my father took it out on and often outraged our family. My father died in poverty 31 years ago when I was 28 years old. When he died, I did not feel sad at all. But, I can have understood and forgiven him little by little for 31 years.

I had rented other's house for a month and concentrated on my breath there all day for 3 weeks. Although I had done so 5 times until 1995, I could gotten rid of neither the fever of my depression nor my stickiness about my old bitter trouble. Furthermore, I had been apt to take it out on my family (wife and 4 children) the same as my father did.

It is easy to erase your sticky immaterial like a soft jelly in your muscle, but it is very difficult to erase your sticky immaterial within your bones like a strong tenacious snake. I have been fighting against this strong tenacious snake since 2 years ago.

It is very difficult to erase the fever of depression, too. It took me 5-6 hours every night from 1995 to 1997 to erase 80-90% of my fever of depression. Every night, I concentrated silently on my fever of depression whose color was black red brown, I puffed it out patiently together with my exhalation. My depressed emotion about my bitter love trouble of 33 years ago had lived in my fever of depression persistently. I had remembered my bitter love trouble naturally for 1-2 hours during 33 years.

I often felt so painful that I wanted to give up puffing out the fever of depression about my bitter love trouble. Whenever I was puffing out the fever of depression about my old bitter trouble, I felt as if I soaked myself in a bathtub of warm urine. I carried through puffing out my fever of depression for 5-6 hours every night during 2 years patiently by all means. Now, I seldom remember my bitter love trouble.

In the universe, there is not the fever of depression such as steam of warm urine.

Furthermore, since then I have become very sensitive to the fever of depression that belongs to other people, domestic animals, dog, garden tree, potted plants, or the crops. Almost whenever the immaterial fiber or third attention of man or of woman touches me, I feel as if I were touched by a mop soaked in warm urine. At that time, I think I like more the bloodthirstiness of don Juan Matus than other's fever of depression. There was not the fever of depression in don Juan Matus' bloodthirstiness when don Juan Matus got angry like a strong tiger. Don Juan Matus (who is floating in the universe as an inorganic-being) understands me and smiles.

The picture that is drawn by Mr. Yamagata, a Japanese painter is very popular in U.S.A. I think his picture is colorful and beautiful, but I feel some fever of depression and some stickiness have remained in his picture. I think the feeling of his picture is that of inner space of the earth. The feeling of color in the far distant universe is cooler, drier, and glossier. Far distant universe has neither stickiness nor the fever of depression.

As for me, the complaints about my parents and my old bitter trouble had been the second or the third biggest origin of stickiness for long years. They had been depriving me of joy, peace and ability for long years. They had made me unhealthy, stupid and inefficient for long years. They had let me fall into heavy oil sea or hell

I could not have confirmed the existence of my third attention until I began to read Mr. Carlos Castaneda's books since 7 years ago. My female inorganic ally visited me twice shaking the ceiling of my home-town house when I was 10 or 11 year old boy. In those days when I played a baseball as a pitcher in the playground of the elementary school, I could know every ball's destination and direction 3 feet in front of every batter. Before a batter swung a bat, I could know where to go about every ball correctly which I threw. It lasted all day for two days. I was so frighten that I ran away to my house thinking why?

When I played a baseball as a pitcher, my third attention shot out from my body to a batter and made me know the destination and direction of every ball beforehand all day. Then, my third attention brought me silent knowledge. The subtler the third attention is, the more efficient it is. It can be compared to smoke in a treasure-chest. In most cases one who has active useful third attention can not be conscious of its shooting out from one's body. One thinks something special and mysterious has worked on for one. One may think such something is God or a good fortune. Before one's third attention begins to shoot out from one's body and work on for one, the stop of the internal dialogue and peculiar inner silence have to happen to one even when one moves, works, plays, talks, hears, eats, sniffs, touch, sings, pray, goes to stool, and makes love. Because I threw a ball without internal dialogue, I could handle my third attention. In such a case, I emitted something from my body, sank into inner silence and fused with the energy of the surroundings. I can succeed in concentrating on my action, my thought or imagination. I feel as if I were melted. Peculiar silence and peculiar happy lucky feeling governs my surroundings. If I look into my body, I can recognize my body is burning beautifully, silently, coolly and violently. In most cases, I can beckon the spirit and fuse with the spirit.

As I became in my late teens, I became very sensitive to the bad relationship between my father and my mother. They often quarreled and talked about their divorce. My father often outraged my family involving me. I often thought I tried to disappear from my hometown house, but I stopped. I thought I had to be patient in my hometown house in Kyoto Prefecture in Japan until I graduated from high school.

I entered Osaka City University in Japan and left my hometown house in Kyoto Prefecture. My grandmother living with my parents committed suicide by throwing herself to the river before I graduated from it. I barely graduated from it earning money for myself and began to live in Tokyo, Japan Capital City at the age of 22. Just after I began to live in Tokyo, I experienced the bitter love trouble.

The complaints about my parents and my bitter love trouble had been giving me much stickiness and deprived me of joy, happy feeling, peace, inner silence so that I had made my third attention almost dead and useless. My third attention had been confined to the dirty stickiness of my body and of my aura, and could not have moved freely. I had remembered the complaints about my parents and my bitter love trouble for 2-4 hours everyday for about 30 years. I had been foolish enough to waste time on the destructive for 2-4 hours for long years. When I rented a house in mountains at the age of 45 about 14 years ago, I concentrated only on my breath all day for 3 weeks. Then, something like a pouch of sticky bloody pus exploded suddenly in my body. A pouch of sticky bloody pus was full of my complaint about my parents. Since then, my complaint about my parents has almost disappeared.

At the age of 50 about 9 years ago, I rented a house at a fishing harbor and concentrated on my breath all day for 3 weeks doing 3-week fasting. Then, I felt the part just above the center of my eyebrows collapsed and a small hole appeared there. A small hole's diameter was about an inch. So, I could begin to feel spacious and less sticky. I felt as if I went out of a harbor to a vast ocean for the first time. I could begin to be engulfed by manlier atmosphere. This part of the forehead is called a sex organ or a white noble bird in Indian Yoga, too. I can feel my sex energy ascents to it and feel the smell of my sex energy from it. I think my third attention has barely begun to work on again since then after an interval of 40 years. Sometimes, the idea that glances off me is realized.

The third attention is very strange and odd. When my third attention works on very well and the ideas that glanced off me have been realized 10-20 times in succession, I feel weird and fearful. When the ideas about society and big disasters that glanced off me have been realized 10-20 times in succession, I feel as if I become the almighty God. I feel more weird and fearful. I want to throw the almighty God away. I want to throw my third attention away. When my third attention does not work on at all, I fail 10-20 times in succession. Then, I feel missing my third attention. I hope my third attention will work on for me again.

When my third attention works on well, my aura and my physical body are not sticky. I do not feel I get stuck or depressed. Then, I feel happy, healthy, satisfied, light, peaceful and silent. To be sure, good complexion, good appetite, good bowl movement and subtle breath have to have happened to me before my third attention works on well for me. If you do not need your third attention, you had better feel stuck, unhappy, sad, dull, hateful, cynical, unhealthy, unsatisfied, depressed, turbulent and foggy as possible. Furthermore, you had better make every effort to make bad complexion, bad appetite, bad bowl movement, bad sleeping, bad sex, rough breath happen to you. If you want to suspend your third attention temporarily, you had better eat a little more or smoke or remember unhappy, unhealthy people or stop going to stool or make unpleasant love or lack in sleeping or not practice any body exercise.

When we shoot out our immaterial fibers from our bodies, we can not be conscious of shooting out them. The third attention is much subtler and is at much more super high speed than immaterial fiber. It is very difficult for us to be conscious of shooting out the third attention from our bodies. In most cases, we can confirm its existence by the effects which have been brought about by it.

Our third attention can both fly into the far distant universe and bring about any effect within a second or 2 seconds. It is apt to do anything subtly, faintly, swiftly, sweetly, softly, smartly, silently, relentlessly, strongly, perfectly, kindly. Such a way can not be explained by words. The mood of such a way resembles that of the universe and of the spirit. By the way, the universe kills those who do not deserve to enter into them in the same way. The universe heals those who are loved by it in the same way, too.

To be able to confirm the existence of the third attention and handle it, you had better concentrate on your inhalation and exhalation all day for 3 weeks. You will be able to stop your breath automatically after you concentrate on your breath all day for 2 weeks. Then, you will be able to lose most of your stickiness and your third attention will appear from your body.

Furthermore, you had better stare at a star which you like for 30 minutes-an hour every night to be able to confirm the existence of your third attention. Your third attention is so fast that it can fly to a 2 billion light year distant star within a second or 2 seconds. The earth is too small for you to be in practice in your third attention. So, it is difficult for you to be conscious of the moment you shoot out it to an object on the earth. But, you can be conscious of the moment you shoot out it to a star. You feel you shoot out your third attention to a star. If you shoot out your third attention to the space between two stars, you feel as if you shot out a gun or cannon shell to the universe from your body.

Staring at a star you like, you can be conscious of shooting out your third attention to a star. Your third attention can reach most stars within a second or 2 seconds. You can realize that you can catch on a star. Some day, you may be surprised to find that most stars are like ghosts. They have died and vanished. Only the spinning lights of theirs are flying to the earth. Many kinds of the spirits will descend to you from the places of the universe that you stare at, too. They will descend to you like a big waterfall, shower, powder, falling star, gun, cannon shell, big balloon, soap bubble, cylinder, emptiness, or something. They push or pull you. If you are weak or are not deserved to the spirit, you will be fainted or killed.

Furthermore, you will be apt to carry your thought, voice, feeling, smell and sense of touch on your third attention to the universe, any place or any human-being. The spirit floating in the universe finds your offering to the universe, descends to you immediately, and helps you. The noble degree of the spirit descending to you is proportionate to the noble degree of your thought, voice, feeling, smell, sense of touch that you send to the universe.

Most of the universe is in absolute zero (-273.15 c°). Some parts of the universe are in high temperature. Some part of the universe is full of sulfuric acid.

A sticky organism, such as a human being, animal, plant, or devil that lives on the surface of the earth or in inner space, can not live in the harsh environment of the universe. Huna magic in Hawaii says "the meanings for MANA (divine power) are to branch out, and skill and arid, desert" "MA means to fade away, the syllable NA means calmed, quieted, pacified" "MANA (divine power) was symbolized by water and fire"(Mastering Your Hidden Self by Mr. Serge King). I think water means absolute zero and fire means high temperature in the universe. The harsh universe shuts out sticky organism so that it is sacred and powerful. Your third attention is made from your physical body that is a sticky organism. So, at the beginning, it is difficult for your third attention to break through the sticky warm inner space and enter into the extreme hotness or coldness of the universe. If we fall into a furnace, we will vanish immediately and faint purple smoke will ascent for a split second.

To absorb inorganic energy from a stone, you had better stare at a stone or a rock which you like for 30 minutes-an hour everyday, and put stones around your bed and your house.

I recommend that you put a set of a piece of red granite, a piece of gray granite, a piece of marble, a piece of black-tourmaline on the four corners of your bed or of your body. Ancient Egyptian Pyramids at Giza are made of these four kinds of stones. A coffin in a pyramid is made of a big piece of red granite. Mr.Edgar Cayce said that a black stone was put on the top of a pyramid and pieces of black stones were sprinkled around the coffin in the pyramid. You had better absorb and feel inorganic energy from these stones around you. You may feel a piece of gray granite make you cool. Gray granite makes your stickiness and the fever of depression decrease.

When I attended Tensegrity workshop in summer in 1998 in the suburb of Los Angels, I was staring at the rocks of the low mountain every at sunrise and sunset. At the last sunrise, an old dignified strong woman (floating between the mountain and me) appeared saying "you have understood, haven't you? ", and gave me dry red energy. When I came back to Japan, I tried to throw up it to the universe from my body. It broke through sticky inner space easily. Furthermore, I could have cleaned up the sky above my house using it, too.

Many kinds of sticky, feverish, cold or numb immaterial clouds are floating above our head and our houses. They are running sticky, feverish, cold or numb energy into our bodies so as to weaken or kill us. To set ourselves free or cure diseases of ours or of others, we have to cut the pipe between us and such a cloud. When we can cut a pipe, such a cloud breaks. Then, something like sticky soft excrement suddenly pours down to us or a devil living in such a cloud falls off. Or, to cut such a pipe, we had better spin our bodies stopping the movement of the energy around our bodies. Then, something sticky will spatter once for all violently.

The third attention is so subtle and faint that it can be compared to a smoke in a treasure-chest. But it is very strong and nimble. An evangelist and pastor, Mr.Mahesh Chavda can handle his subtle and faint third attention. He has All Nations Church in North Carolina in U.S.A. I saw in August in 1999 in Japan that his dry third attention was very strong and could invade into anything immediately although it seemed to be very subtle, faint, weak and light. I could believe that he could revive a dead child in 1985 and cure the 3000 blind at once in Africa.

You had better begin to know the existence of a smoke in a treasure-chest and open a treasure-chest. You have to make a smoke go to any place you want, return to a treasure-chest at any time you want intentionally, and close a treasure-chest.

To strengthen and purify a smoke as possible, you have to make a smoke catch on many kinds of the spirits which are more beautiful, drier, glossier, cooler, sweeter, stronger, swifter, nimbler, kinder, softer, more relentless, fiercer. Although the spirits may hate a smoke which tries to catch on the spirits and may try to explode a smoke to death immediately, you have to challenge at your peril to strengthen and purify a smoke (your third attention).

When you have some big complaint or when dirty energy bodies of others and devils stick to or enter into you, you will become sticky and lose your awareness. They can break your direction signals so that you will become at a loss what to do or how to do or where to go. You will able to concentrate on nothing. You will have nothing to do with enthusiasms. You will be taken over by some big complaint, dirty energy bodies of others or devils and become unhappy, unhealthy, inefficient. Then, you had better remember the feeling of the common denominator about all opposite sexes whom you have loved in detail as much as possible to shut out your big complaint, dirty energy bodies of others or devils.

In this respect, opposite sexes on the earth are quite strange and odd. They are both big obstacles and big benefactors for us to become happy, healthy, and efficient. Opposite sexes are like powerful drugs that are both poisons and medicines for us.

Happy, healthy, successful people are apt to make their third attention work on for them unconsciously and keep on being happy, healthy, and successful. But, they will be at a loss what to do when they have made their third attention dead and useless. In most cases, they do not know how to revive their third attention. They will be disgraced miserably in 3-5 years. So, they had better read my book and revive their third attention. They had better remember and recover the feeling of dryness, of rustling, of not getting stuck, of not getting depressed.

Unhappy, unhealthy, unfortunate people have gotten stuck or depressed by stickiness, fever of depression, coldness or numbness, and made their third attention dead and useless. They have not made their third attention work on for them at all, so they can not understand what I have written about the third attention, stickiness, immaterial fiber, concentration, peculiar happy feeling, the spirit, body-response in my book at all and ignore them.

As for me, I could not have understood the third attention and had ignored it completely if I had not concentrated on my breath all day for 3 weeks 5 times by 9 years ago and if my third attention had not worked on for me during playing a baseball all day for 2 days at the age of 10-11. As a result, I could not have understood Mr. Carlos Castaneda books, Cabala, Ancient Egyptian Pyramid Text, The

Emerald-Tablet of Thoth-The-Atlantean, Yoga Sutra and so on at all. I think all of them try to teach us how to get rid of stickiness, how to cure or prevent depression, how to become happy, healthy, efficient, how to burn the fire from within our bodies, how to shoot out our immaterial fibers or third attention to an object from our bodies, how to succeed in concentrating on something that we like, how to be conscious of the third attention, how to handle it, how to contact the spirit, how to fly into the universe freely, and how to live in the universe for long years as an inorganic being.

Danger can erase stickiness, too. Animals in a safe zoo, domestic animals, pets, garden trees, potted plants and the crops have much stickiness, but wild animals and wild plants which live in a harsh struggle for existence have little stickiness. So, you had better run a risk at your peril in your life to erase your stickiness.

Sometimes, you had better act desperately about your work and hobby. Sometimes, you had better enter into a dangerous place. Sometimes you had better venture your life, physical body, post or all your money at your peril.

Sticky unhealthy-unhappy-inefficient people or depressed people hate a danger, desperate action, and dangerous place, but rustling healthy-happy-successful people like them and can enjoy them. Even the former US president, Geoge Bush enjoyed a dangerous sky diving in spite of his old age in summer in 1999. You had better like a danger and adventure to shut out stickiness, too. Uneducated people are apt to be healthier, happier, or more successful than educated people because uneducated people like a danger and adventure more than educated people so that they have less stickiness. If you become less sticky, you can release your immaterial fiber or third attention from the stickiness, shoot out your immaterial fiber or third attention to an outside object, judge it accurately, control it, succeed in concentrating on it, and attain happy lucky feeling, inspiration, health and supernatural power through the success of concentration.

If you want to cure or prevent depression, you had better live like not as an animal in a safe zoo but as an animal in a dangerous Africa plain.

If you prefer to live like an animal in a safe zoo, you will be safe for a while and begin to become sticky. As a result, you begin to have bad complexion, make your fire within your body go out, get stuck and depressed, can not shoot out your immaterial fiber or third attention, can not judge it accurately, can not control it, can not concentrate on it, can not attain happy lucky feeling, inspiration, health or supernatural power through the success of concentration and can not realize what you imagine or think of. Then, you become unhappy-unhealthy-inefficient.

If you live like an animal in a dangerous African plain, you will become less sticky, and become alert and strong. Even in a zoo, danger and struggle seem to be essential for animals to live long. The curator of some zoo said "If I make a male giraffe live together with 10 female giraffes, a male giraffe will die of disease soon. If I make 2 male giraffes live together with 10 female giraffes, 2 male giraffes will not die of disease soon but live long although they fight about 10 female giraffes and always injure their necks each other because of their fight".

I want to live and die like a wild animal in a dangerous Africa plain. If I suffer from depression, I will neither go to doctors nor take the medicine of anti-depression. If I suffer from cancer, I will neither take medical treatment nor operation. I want to die while walking or working. In such a respect, I have written this book. If you do not agree to my thoughts, you had better stop reading my book and live like an animal in a safe zoo or a male giraffe living together with 10 female giraffes. I hope only the readers who agree to my thoughts will read my book as many as possible and take advantage of some content of my book at their perils.

## Hunt and multiply various good feelings

The Scriptures say "Kingdom is coming. Repent!". Repent is to change your bad feeling. Happy good feeling is power. Happy good feeling can give you a supernatural power, cure diseases and change your surroundings for better.

Happy good feeling is proportionate to (1)doing some proper body-exercise such as constricting anus 100 times and denting navel 100 times everyday at least for 10 years patiently (2)the degree of your internal organ's strength (3)the ability to erase your dirty stickiness of your body and of your aura (4)your body's fire's strength and beauty (5)the degree of good complexion (6)firm and soft strong abdomen, waist, hip, buttock, inside of thigh and outside of thigh (7)the rotation of your body's vortexes (8)the ability to stop your internal dialogue (9)the ability to beckon inner silence (10)the ability to shoot out your immaterial fiber or third attention to an outside object, judge it accurately and control it (11)succeed in concentrating on an outside object and attain happy lucky feeling, inspiration, health and supernatural power through the success of concentration (12)the ability to realize what you imagine or think of (13)the ability to make friends with danger or death (14)the ability to act, talk and see with abandon, largess and humor to beckon the spirit (15)the ability to talk, pray, preach or sing from the bottom of your abdomen with abandon, largess and humor (16)the ability to stop your breath automatically (17)the frequency of fasting (18)the ability to find power-spot (19)the ability to stare at something with the middle of your eyebrows broadened (20)the ability to follow your body-response.

Please, test how much power and good feeling you have now before you begin to read Hunt and multiply various good feeling of Part 7. Test (1)when you think about a good point of someone (who is at a different place) for a few seconds-30 minutes, someone will send you a present ,invite you to dinner or call you in 3 days although you do not ask someone to do so (2)when you think about a good point of someone ( who is at a different place) for a few seconds-30 minutes, someone will recover from the serious illness or will get well (3)when you stare at a stray cat, it will suddenly lies on its back in front of you and show its abdomen to show you honor.

If none of them happens to you, you have neither power nor happy good feeling at all. You have to recognize "I have given poison to someone and a stray cat, or can have given nothing to them. I am unhealthy-unhappy-inefficient now". In such a case, please, read my book many times and recover power and happy good feeling. If you are a big man or founder or enterpriser, you had better retire amicably before you are miserably disgraced.

If two thirds of (1)(2)(3) or all (1)(2)(3) happen to you, you have power and happy good feeling. You have to recognize "I have given something good to someone or a stray cat. I am healthy-happy-efficient". In such a case, you do not have to read my book or had better read it once to prepare against the future loss of your power and of your happy good feeling. If you are a big man, founder or enterpriser, you do not have to retire and had better be active in the front lines.

To cure or prevent depression and become healthy-happy-efficient, you had better follow your body-response to your surroundings. Goethe said "we are tricked not by body-response but by reason". But, body-response has not happened to most of us because it has been broken by our stickiness, complaints, lack of body-exercise, bad abdomens-hips and so on. So, most of us can neither find nor catch what gives health-happiness-efficiency to us. What can give health-happiness-efficiency to us is power. Power is special good feeling, mood, atmosphere, another world and time.

Most of us have been confined to one or two bad feelings which are sticky, feverish, cold, numb, depressed, angry, hateful, irritated, self-pity, guilty, fearful, gloomy, dull, cynical, stubborn, restless, busy, sly or timid. Such a feeling is the core of unhealthy-unhappy-inefficient individual and home. That is to say, in such a case, our immaterial fibers or third attention are confined to dirty energy (something like heavy oil, sludge, mud, sewage) of our bodies and can not be shot out from it to an outside object. That is to say, we can not concentrate on an outside object. As a result, we can not see an outside object through accurately and can neither control nor change it freely. If we are confined to such a bad feeling for long time, we will made our immaterial fibers or third attention almost dead and will become unhealthy-unhappy-inefficient. Unfortunately, we will have forgotten another special good feeling if we have been confined to the bad feeling for more than 6 months.

To break from the bad feeling, you had better remember(1) the common denominators about all opposite sexes whom you have loved (aura's color, smell, sense of touch, voice, temperature of all opposite sexes in detail as possible whom you have loved) (2) the happiest scene in your life.

Furthermore, to break from the bad feeling, you had better imagine (3)spring, east wind in the morning, light spring breeze, morning, sprout, adolescence, young virgin, healthy strong liver, healthy strong tendon, good eye, cunning, blue color, primeval tree, rancid smell, twitter, being airy and nimble (4)summer, south wind at night, daytime, luxuriance, youth, healthy strong heart, smell of burning, joy, ruthless, sex appeal, lewdness, activity, grow thick, catch on, swallow up, self-confidence, taking care of somebody, red, fire, riotousness (5)the end of summer, southwest wind in the end of summer, at P.M 2-3, manhood, healthy strong spleen, healthy strong muscle, sweet, yellow, the center of the earth, hidden super-power, hidden big collapse, fragrant smell, chemical reaction, digestion, change ,invasion and adhering, peace (6)autumn, west wind in autumn, at P.M 3-5, the beginning of late life, healthy strong lung, healthy beautiful skin, ripeness, white color, frost, tiger, choice, the sky of autumn, clarity, purification, fishing smell, moderate sadness, genius and insanity, strictness (7)transparency, healthy strong V-spot on the crest of the sternum at the base of your neck, clarity, smooth, seer, the eye of hawk (8)winter, north wind in winter, at noon, late life, healthy strong kidney, healthy strong bones, good ear, stop, death, rest, detachment, black, mother, water, silent voice on the back of the ear, decree, rotten smell, patience, bravery, rushing headlong, originality, arrogance.

Don Juan Matus, the teacher of the late Mr.Carlos Castaneda says in the book with the title-Journey to Ixtlan "Personal power is a feeling. Something like being lucky. Or one may call it a mood", in the book with the title-Power of Silence "You need to be ruthless (of (4)), cunning (of (3)), patient (of (8)) and sweet (of (5)). Ruthless should not be harshness, cunning should not be cruelty, patience should not be negligence, sweetness should not be foolishness"

If you have been confined to the bad feeling for long years (or for several months) and forgotten another special good feeling completely, you had better imagine your bad feeling at the beginning and (1)-(2)-(3)-(4)-(5)-(6)-(7)-(8)-your bad feeling one after another. Then, you had better begin to keep on having the best feeling of these feelings that you have imagined.

The lively you can imagine so, the more easily you can begin to change your dream during dreaming intentionally. The lively you can imagine so, the more easily you can change your surroundings. After you can change your dream during dreaming intentionally, you will begin to change your surroundings, For example, someone around you feels cold in summer when you imagine the coldness of winter in spite of being in summer. If you can imagine the feeling of summer's rain lively in dry season, it will begin to rain in dry season. You had better be able to change the scenes during dreaming intentionally, too. As a result, you can cure your or other disease and can improve your surroundings by imagining good feeling. Furthermore, an angel or the spirit that has the same feeling as that of your good feeling begins to approach you and help you after you threw away bad feeling and begin to have new good feeling. So, you will cure disease and improve your surroundings much more easily.

The spirit that is floating in the universe, inner space or the interior of the earth is approaching you as a gassy energy of special color or a transparent energy. If you can see that the spirit which has good feeling is approaching you, you had better make your immaterial fiber or third attention catch on it.

The spirit sticks its pipe into your physical body or your aura during your dreaming, too. In such a case, you had better grasp both the tip of the pipe and the pipe during your dreaming if you feel better about the feeling of its tip. You can keep on grasping the spirit for longer time than you grasp only its tip. At A.M 3 yesterday, I was aware that the tip of the spirit's pipe stuck in my right eye and flashed in my dream. It had a healthy strong feeling of white and red color. It seemed to have the ability to erase the stickiness or the fever of depression in our bodies. It seemed that I would be able to cure diseases of others by flowing it to others. Its scene was very lively. I thought its scene was not an illusion but a reality. So, I got up immediately, went out of my house, and looked up the sky from which the spirit seemed to shoot out a pipe to me. Then, the flashing energy of the spirit's good feeling descended to me from the sky. The spirit presented me a new different good feeling last night, too.

Imaging good feelings is compared to putting key word into a personal computer. The ability to imagine good feelings is proportionate to the beauty, dryness, gloss, flexibility, activity, and peace of your energy body. These of your energy body are proportionate to your good complexion, rejuvenation, good appetite, good sleeping, good bowel movement, and soft shoulder. These healthy features are proportionate to (1) healthy strong liver-gallbladder, healthy strong heart-a small intestine, a pancreas, the healthy strong spleen-stomach, healthy strong lung-a large intestine, healthy strong V-spot of neck, healthy strong kidney-bladder (2) developing the muscles of abdomen, waist, hip, thigh firmly and softly (getting rid of poor, flabby, fat, or stiff abdomen, waist, hip, thigh) (3) having good spine (4) shutting out opposite sexes without sadness, or pleasant and satisfied sex (5)the ability to stop your breath automatically (6)eating in moderation.

(1)(2)(3)(4)(5) are proportionate to practicing what I have written (body exercise, moderation of life, stroll, not smoking, standard weight, yoga, saving sex energy, concentrating on breath, doing fasting, stare, body exercise of Chinese martial arts, making friends with danger, burning the fire from within body, shooting out immaterial fiber or the third attention to an object and succeeding in concentrating on it, erasing stickiness, following body-response).

Whenever you listen to a lecture of psychology, religion or management, you may be taught many times "You will be healthy-successful if you have a positive thinking and positive self-image". But, in most cases, you will fail to have a positive thinking and positive self-image and fail to realize health and success whenever you try to have such a thinking and self-image.

It is because that dirty energy body of other, devil and your complaints(about opposite sex, health, son or daughter, parents, boss, money, work or post) have made your energy body dirty, sticky, feverish, cold or numb. As a result, the ability to imagine positive thinking and positive self-image has declined.

It can be compared to putting the key word (positive thinking and positive self-image) into a personal computer that has fallen into heavy oil, sludge or sewage. You had better take the personal computer from heavy oil, sludge, sewage, and wash-repair-make it run on electricity. Then, you can put the key word into it and make it work on for you. What I have written (body exercise, moderation of life, stroll, not smoking, standard weight, yoga, saving sex energy, concentrating on breath, doing fasting, stare, body exercise of Chinese martial arts, making friends with danger, burning the fire from within body, shooting out your immaterial fiber or the third attention to an object and succeeding in concentrating on it, erasing stickiness, and following body-response) is compared to taking such a personal computer from heavy oil, sludge, sewage and washing-repairing-making it run on electricity again. So, practicing what I have written, you had better imagine above-mentioned good feelings.

Healthy strong liver can give you the good feeling of cunning and of light spring breeze. Healthy strong heart can give you the good feeling of joy, of self-confidence and of abandon. Healthy strong spleen can give you the good feeling of sweet. Healthy strong lung can give you the good feeling of moderate sadness and of kindness. Healthy strong V-spot of neck give you the good feeling of clarity. Healthy strong kidney can give you the good feeling of patience, of originality and of bravery.

So, you had better cure or strengthen your liver, heart, spleen, lung, V-spot, and kidney by all means, for example by what I have written. There exist close connections through energy pipes between liver and gallbladder, between heart and a small intestine-pancreas, between spleen and stomach, between lung and a large intestine, between kidney and bladder. As a result, to cure or strengthen your liver, heart, spleen, lung, and kidney, you had better cure or strengthen your gallbladder, a small intestine-pancreas, stomach, a large intestine and bladder, too.

Healthy strong liver gives you the feeling of light spring breeze or of a tree's sprout that can relax and seduce other people.

About for 2 weeks after you finish fasting, you can enjoy happy relieved feeling and can imagine lively. For example, you can imagine Brazil lively. If you have come back to U.S.A from Brazil and can tell someone a lively story about your life in Brazil, your third attention or immaterial fiber can go to Brazil and stay there while telling. The way to confirm the working of your third attention or immaterial fiber is to be able to imagine some place, someone, or some place lively. Then, by the grace of your third attention or immaterial fiber, what you imagine is not an illusion but a reality and the result of realization. So, the

Scriptures say "fast and pray". Regrettably, as the pastors of U.S.A become older, they are apt to become fat because of eating too much.

In most cases, such a happy relieved feeling will pass away 2 weeks later after you left a center of fasting. You will begin to eat animal food, animal-protein, much sugar, much salt, drink coffee, alcohol and the water with chlorine, eat or drink the foods or the water boiled in aluminum pot or kettle, eat or drink the foods or water which the constituent parts of plastic soak into, smoke, take the medicine, do not chew well, do not have a stroll, do not some proper exercise, make love so that the dirty stickiness of your body and of your aura will increase again and your happy relieved feeling will pass away. As the result of happy relieved feeling's passing away, you can neither imagine lively nor change your dream freely, so that your third attention or your immaterial fiber is confined to your aura or physical body and stops working on for you again. Then, what you imagine or dream is only an illusion or a dream.

About for 2 weeks after you finish fasting, you can imagine lively. It takes some time for it to be realized. You feel happy when it is realized. There remains some stickiness or the fever of depression in this liveliness.

When you can begin to feel so happier that you want to neither accomplish nor gain anything, some stickiness or some fever of depression in this liveliness is eliminated. You become selfless. Then, what you imagine or think of other people or society or psychic world subtly and lightly without eagerness can be realized only in a few seconds. You feel so weird and fearful when it is realized 10-20 in succession that you never tell proudly what it is realized. You can not begin to have such a super power of imagination as long as you take advantage of a power of imagination to realize your own wishes.

A powerful engine has to be cooled by air or water. If it were not cooled, it will break down, be fired or exploded to pieces. The more powerful a engine is, the more it has to be cooled. Red energy of heart has to be cooled by the cool white fog energy of lung, too. Heart hates excessive hotness. Energetic heart is weakened by excessive hotness, so energetic joyful heart has to be cooled by the sad white energy of lung. To keep on being big men, big men have to have much sadness (kindness, mercy) as well as much joy-ruthless-activity.

Excessive transparent black energy without yellow energy is useless. It only keeps on rushing headlong so recklessly and arrogantly as to suicide. There is the same type of people among us because they only have strong healthy kidneys and do not have strong healthy spleens. They rush headlong, fight and ruin. They have only sticks, and do not have carrots.

Strong healthy spleen emits sweet yellow energy. Sweet yellow energy can lay restrain on excessive black energy's activity which healthy strong kidney has. If we rush headlong sweetly, we can rush headlong without much resistance. It can be compared to the famous saying-the carrot and the stick.

In this respect, most of us had in the childhood (1)the feeling of light spring breeze (beautiful blue energy) (2)the feeling of gloss (beautiful transparent energy) (3)the feeling of sweetness (beautiful yellow energy). But, most of us are apt to have thrown away them since adulthood because of the complaints (about opposite sex, health, son or daughter, parents, boss, work, money, or post). Most of us think "I can believe not in others but only in myself "and become cynical. Throwing away them can be compared to a rusty rifle which has not a trench of barrel, a leaf, a sight line.

In such a case, most of us can not fire a bullet (red energy of heart, white energy of lung, black energy of kidney). Most of us can not shoot out our useful immaterial fibers or the third attentions to an outside object and can not see, judge or control an outside object well. It also can be compared to a machine without lubrication.

Big men, founders, happy-healthy-efficient people are apt not to throw away the feeling of light spring breeze, the feeling of gloss and the feeling of sweet in spite of complaints. Their energies, feelings, atmospheres, behaviors, voices and complexion are light, glossy and sweet. They have such good pheromones or attractions to control others without interests or threat. If they have lost such good pheromones or attractions for long time, they will be disgraced by many attacks of others sooner or later.

But, only the feeling of light spring breeze, the feeling of gloss and the feeling of sweet without the feeling of self-confidence, of abandon, of ruthless, of activity (beautiful red energy of heart)-the feeling of insanity and genius (beautiful white energy of lung)-the feeling of rushing headlong, of bravery (beautiful black energy of kidney) are useless. Only the feeling of light spring breeze, the feeling of gloss and the feeling of sweet can be compared to a rifle without bullets or a teethless tiger and will be looked down upon sooner or later.

Power is the good feeling. To begin to hunt power and the good feelings, and prevent or cure depression, you had better (1)strengthen your various internal organs, become more healthy, and grow at least 10-20 years old younger by doing some proper body-exercise following the life style of long-lived British (2)sometimes turn to bay throwing pride or play the part of blockhead or take anything as it comes (3)do 3-week fasting (4)talk, see or act with abandon, largess and humor and can beckon the spirit (5)stare at something with the middle of eyebrows broadened (6)concentrate on something (7) be able to shoot out your immaterial fiber or your third attention to an outside object from your body ,see it through, control it, succeed in concentrating on it, and attain happy lucky feeling, inspiration, health and supernatural power through the success of concentration (If your immaterial fiber or third attention is compelled to be confined to your physical body or your aura, you will feel irritated, self-pity, inferiority complex, guilty, depressed, stuck, indecisive, fearful ) (8)be able to stop your breath automatically (9)become on the point of dying or make friends with danger (10)find and stay a power-spot (11)cure the trouble of spine (12)follow your body-response (13) remember or imagine beautiful strong feeling's scenes (14)eat acid foods to strengthen liver, eat bitter foods to strengthen heart, eat sweet foods to strengthen spleen, eat hot foods to strengthen lung or eat salty foods to strengthen kidney-eat a well-balanced diet (15)absorb beautiful strong energy from stones, stars, and the spirits (16)be presented beautiful strong energy by the spirits (17)listen to the voices of healthy-happy-efficient people and the voices of founders, of big men, of pioneers and of enterprisers who have not been disgraced and have not been proud or careless (18)listen to the voices which are uttered by the central energy pipe of physical body or are uttered from abdomen (19)listen to the silent voice(the voice of God, voice without voice on the back of left ear).

To hunt bigger power as possible, you had better hunt various better feelings as possible by all means. Above-mentioned ways to hunt power and the good feeling are just examples.

Don't be satisfied with one beautiful strong color energy of good feeling. You had better search for more beautiful and stronger same color energies of better feeling as possible. Furthermore, you had better search for beautiful strong different color energies of good feeling as possible.

Don Juan Matus says "(most of) our fellow men are black magicians. And whoever is with them is a black magician on the spot. Think for a moment. Can you deviate from the path that your fellow men have lined up for you? And if you remain with them, your thoughts and your actions are fixed forever in their terms. That is a slavery. The warrior, on the other hand, is free from all that" "Freedom is expensive, but the price is not impossible to pay. So, fear your captors, your masters. Don't waste your time and your power fearing freedom"-Tales of Power.

"The world of people goes up and down and people go up and down with their world; warriors have no business following the ups and downs of their fellow men"-The Second Ring of Power.

"The recommendation for warriors is not to have any material things on which to focus their power, but to focus it on the spirit, on the true

flight into the unknown, not on trivialities. Everyone who wants to follow the warriors path has to rid himself of the compulsion to possess
and hold onto things"-The Eagle's Gift.

The etymology of "sin" is to miss the target. To miss the target is to
concentrate not on good feeling (involving the feeling of the spirit) but
on bad feeling. To concentrate on bad feeling is to become stuck,
depressed, irritated, foggy or powerless. To become powerless is to
become unhealthy-unhappy-inefficient. So, change your feeling if you
have followed the bad feeling (such as heavy oil sea, sludge, mud or
sewage) for long time. The Scriptures say "The Kingdom (heaven, the
spirit) is coming to you. Repent! ". The etymology of "Repent!" is to
change your feeling.

# Part 6 Follow comfortable body-response

To cure or prevent and become healthy-happy-efficient, you had better follow your comfortable body-response to the surroundings. Get rid of poor, flabby, fat, or stiff abdomen, waist, hip, and thigh. This is a founder's, pioneer's or master's way of life. It could cure the trouble of my spine, too. Goethe. the famous German dramatist (1749-1832) said "We are tricked not by body-response but by reason".

You can shoot out your immaterial fiber or third attention to the outside object from your body and succeed in concentrating on the outside object easily to which your comfortable body response happen. Furthermore, you can attain much better body-response and happier luckier feeling the moment you can shoot out your immaterial fiber or third attention to the outside object and succeed in concentrating on the outside object easily to which your comfortable body response happen. As a result, you can cure or prevent depression and become healthier-happier-more efficient.

The trouble of my spine had tortured me from the age of 31 to the age of 56 because it had kept on causing the stiff lamp of my under-belly and my frequent urination. By following my body-responses obediently, I could have cured them for 4 years since the age of 52. I had ventured to do anything about which my body-response signaled comfort. They had not been cured by medical treatments and so on at all for long years. I think I should have died of bladder cancer already if I could not have cured them by following my body-response.

Part 6-Follow comfortable body-response shows the examples of my body responses. Furthermore, Part 6-body-response is how to cure the trouble of my spine, the stiff lamp of my underbelly and my frequent urination following my body-responses. Buddha taught the same way in India 2500 years ago for us to be able to become healthy, happy and efficient.

I think that the first or the second biggest origin of depression, paralysis, heart disease, or cancer is the trouble of spine or the complaint about opposite sex, son, daughter, parent, boss, work, money and post.

Especially, the trouble of spine gives us pangs, internal organ's lump and stiff shoulder. It deprives us of peace, inner silence, joy, happy feeling and efficiency. It always makes us irritated or depressed and makes our blood pressure high. When we quarrel with a wife, child, colleague or chief, we fall down easily after the age of 45 because our blood pressure rises up to 180-200 suddenly. At first, we can sit up within 30 seconds-2 hours. In 2-3 years since then, we will fall down completely.

Furthermore, cancer is apt to happen to the internal organ that has lamp. An internal organ is connected with spine through autonomic nerve. So, the internal organ in front of the disordered part of spine begins to become weak, has lamp and cancer is apt to happen to it.

Violent sports (soccer, Rugby, and so on), intense exercise, dash, dance, golf, yoga, long meditation, or accident is apt to injure spine.

Furthermore, the weakening of the back's muscle and of abdomen's muscle makes the bone of spine turn aside. Spine is supported by the muscle of the back and of abdomen. When we become older than 50 years old, we are apt to begin to be suffering from the gap of our spine if we have not keep on strengthening the muscle of the back and of abdomen. Stroll (one-hour everyday) and the reverse movement of body (for example, Tensegrity) can strengthen the muscle of the back and of abdomen.

When no problem is with spine, most of us are so careless or so proud of good fortune that most of us say we are too busy to strengthen the muscle of the back and of abdomen. Most of us go anywhere not on foot but by car. Once we begin to be suffering from the trouble of spine, we can not get well easily. The success rate of the operation is not so high. We will be half paralyzed as the result of the operation's failure.

As I have written, the complaints about both my parents and my old bitter love trouble had given me much stickiness for 20-34 years. This stickiness had deprived me of joy, peace and ability and made me unhealthy-unhappy-inefficient. Furthermore, my spine was injured by a woman massager of a sauna bath in Tokyo 28 years ago when I was about 31 years old. In those days, I worked for a newspaper as a journalist.

The sauna bath permitted the last customers sleep on the stands of in Japan. It took me one hour to come back to my apartment from Tokyo. Although I had the wife, I felt tiresome to come back to my apartment when I drank alcohol. After I drank alcohol almost every night, I went to the sauna bath at dead of night and was given a massage. In most cases after a massage, I slept on the stand of massage until the morning. Almost every night, I made a woman massager step my spine.

Then, I tried to get up at my apartment in the morning, but I could not get up because of the pangs of my spine. I could not get up for a week. I felt the pangs whenever I inhaled and exhaled my breath. I felt as if I cried for the pangs of my spine when I went to stool.

A week later, I barely got up and went to Kyoto to cure the gap of my spine. The professional cured the gap of my spine by his fingers and eliminated the pangs of my spine.

But, since then, the subtle unpleasant lamp had happened to my underbelly. It had caused my frequent urination, too. The subtle unpleasant lamp of my underbelly and my frequent urination had kept on torturing me and making me irritated for 25 years.

After 1.5 year impotence, I still felt as if an arrow had pierced my underbelly

For one and half a years since then, I had become impotent in spite of the age of 31-32. I could make ** with my wife because of conditioned reflex movement (?), but I could not make ** with other young women by all means. I can remember a young woman teased me about my impotence. She said "Hey, try, try"giving a wry smile. Such an impotence had been cured unconsciously.

It is regrettable that the pangs of my spine had happened to me for a week still every year from the age of 31 to the age of 56 when I carried something heavy. The subtle unpleasant lamp of my underbelly and my frequent urination had continued almost everyday persistently, too. I felt as if an arrow or a few thorns had kept on piercing my underbelly or as if I had kept on wearing wet underpants. Furthermore, I had been feeling the hangover of urine. I had urinated too often everyday from the age of 32 to the age of 56.

As I have written, my third attention has barely begun to work on for me again since the part just above the center of my eyebrows collapsed at the age of 50. But, my third attention worked on for me only when little problem was with my spine, the lamp of my underbelly or my frequent urination.

The pangs of my spine could have been eliminated by hanging my body from the instrument for body (hanging for about 2-3 minutes everyday for a week). But, I could have eliminated neither the subtle unpleasant lamp of my underbelly nor my frequent urination for long years. They had made me irritated. They had made me have a terrible temper. I had sometimes lost my temper with my 3 daughters, a son and my wife, and outraged them. I had been neither a good father nor a good husband. Thank God, none of my daughters and a son have not become delinquents.

I had been minutely examined at many big hospitals. Nothing had been problem in medical respects. When I insisted on the complaint about my subtle unpleasant lamp of my underbelly and my frequent urination persistently, I was diagnosed with autonomic imbalance. Then, the doctor gave me medicine for autonomic imbalance. I drank it, but it was not effective for me at all.

Acupuncture and moxibustion could cure my subtle unpleasant lamp and my frequent urination only for a few days. They relapsed easily. I had tried many folk medicines, but they had not been effective for me at all. Body exercise of yoga, fasting and meditation had been little effective for me, too.

All was lost. I often thought I would pay as much money as possible if some one could cure my unpleasant lamp and my frequent urination.

I have written in Part 5-Erase your bad stickiness and multiply various good feeling as follows. "When I rented a house in mountains at the age of 45 about 14 years ago, I concentrated only on my breath everyday for 3 weeks. Then, something like a pouch of sticky bloody pus exploded suddenly in my body. A pouch of sticky bloody pus was full of my complaint about my parents. Since then, my complaint about my parents has almost disappeared".

This pouch of sticky bloody pus had been living in the unpleasant lamp of my underbelly. Although the pouch of sticky bloody pus had been eliminated, there had still existed the unpleasant lamp and my frequent urination.

At the age of 51 about 8 years ago, I urinated so often that the crotches of my pants turned to be brown because of my urine leak. I urinated every quarter of an hour and urinated only a little. I took the pants to a laundry, but a laundry could not eliminate the brown of my pants. So, I fired about 20 business suits whose pants turned to be brown heavily at my garden.

Furthermore, the lamp of my underbelly had become stiffer. I felt as if it had been a stone. I often wished I could have gouged the unpleasant lamp of my underbelly by a sharp straight razor. I often felt I would die of bladder-cancer. Because hospitals had been undependable for me, I had not gone to hospital in those days. In those days, the bladder-cancer might have happened to me already.

Such a symptom continued for a year. At the age of 52, I took the express train (Sinctu Line of JR) to the back of Japan. When I glanced at the mountain near Karuizawa. the most famous summer resort in Japan, I felt relieved and relaxed again. Whenever I glanced at the mountain through the window of the train since the age of 35, my body felt relieved and relaxed. I wondered why? I looked at the map and could find a hot spring in the mountain whose nearest station is Yokogawa station. So, at last, I got off the train at Karuizawa station, changed the train, and came back to Yokogawa station.

It took me about half an hour to reach a Japanese-style hotel in the hot spring by the hotel's station wagon. The landlord drove the station wagon along a treacherous path that had steep narrow up-slope, many loops and almost perpendicular cliff. I sweated a little with fear and was excited with his dangerous drive. There was only one Japanese-style hotel (Kintokan, TEL 0273-95-3851) in the hot spring almost at the top of the mountain. It had been serviced with electricity recently.

I had a leisurely bath of the hotel. I was submerged up to my neck in the white lukewarm water. I went out of the water and began to wash my body. I drank a few cups of the white lukewarm water, too. It was a marvel that I felt my head became relieved and relaxed while washing my head with the white lukewarm water of the hot spring. I felt the white lukewarm water was erasing both the stickiness and the fever of depression in my head. Furthermore, I saw a white light began to radiate in my head.

When I came back to my room of the hotel, I looked into my head closing my eyes. The white light was still radiating. I went out of the hotel, I looked down from there at the tops of other mountains. Then, the tops of other mountains radiated white lights, too.

I stayed one night (about 80 dollars) and came back to my house. Then, I felt the stiff lamp of my underbelly like a stone barely twiddled and became fluid a little. The white lukewarm water decreased the frequency of my frequent urination, too. Hospital, body-exercise, yoga, fasting, meditation, concentrating on my breath, folk medicine had little effect to cure the lamp of my underbelly and my frequent urination, so I was very pleased to find for the first time that a hot spring was effective for them.

Next week, I went to this hot spring again to cure them. I stayed for 2 days on weekdays. I felt my head became relieved and relaxed again while washing my head with the white lukewarm water of the hot spring. I felt the white lukewarm water was erasing both the stickiness and the fever of depression in my head again. Furthermore, I felt a white light radiated in my head .The lamp of my underbelly became more fluid and softer, and the frequency of my frequent urination decreased more. Since then, I had been to this hot spring about 10 times.

Only a few or one guest stayed at the hotel weekdays and about 10-20 guests stayed on weekend. I told the landlord "Your hot spring is very effective for me". I told him "I can feel something special about it". He taught this area was the more famous hot spring and summer resort than Karuizawa about 100 years ago.

Many big men in the revolution of Meiji times and big merchants had their cottages there. Mr.Hirobumi Ito had a cottage there who was a big man in the revolution of Meiji times and the prime minister when Japan won China. All of such cottages had been destroyed by big typhoons because this area was the path of big typhoons. Only this landlord's hotel has been saved. Mr. Kaisyu Katu who was a big man in the revolution of Meiji times often visited the landlord's hotel to cure his piles. His short poem has been engraved on the stone in the hotel's garden.

In Meiji times, Japan broke the feudal system and became a modern state. Small poor Japan won big China and big Russia. In those days, it was said "the bigger defect he has, the bigger man he is. A timid sober man is not worthy to talk about". Most ministers of Meiji Government were in twenties. At cabinet councils, most ministers insisted on so violently that they were often on the brink of exchanging blows or flinging chairs.

In the first place, Mr. kaisyu Katu had the vice of making ** with his house's maids one after another, so that his wife said she would not be buried beside his tomb when she died. Mr.Kaisyu Katu often had a narrow escape when he was about to be assassinated by a strong swordsman. Mr. Kaisyu Katu threw away his sword and squatted down cross-legged in front of the strong swordsman saying "Wait, I will be killed by you silently". A strong swordsman could not kill the man who decided to be killed silently without fear. In such a way, he often still had a life. He said "Man should have patience with his bad reputation for 10 years. Disregarding the thoughts of other people, man should do what he believes. 10 years later, other people will change their thoughts and respect such a man". How about Mr. Clinton, the president of U.S.A?

There are many hot springs around Tokyo, the capital of Japan. Big men of Meiji times had big power. They could have cottages or villas at any hot spring around Tokyo. Such big men prefer the hot spring in the mountain near Karuizawa (about one and half an hours by express train from Tokyo) and had cottages there because they recognized the special effect of the hot spring's white lukewarm water.

I think their heads must have become relieved and relaxed while washing their heads with the white lukewarm water of the hot spring. I think they felt white lights radiated in their heads. I think the hot spring eased their tiredness that was caused by administering new poor small Japan.

If our lungs are healthy and not taken over by the stickiness of our complaint, of other people's dirty energy bodies, or of devils, our lungs can radiate white lights and shoot out strong white immaterial fibers to catch on an object. White energy can cure disease of ours and of others easily, shut out devils, and has strong attack-power like a tiger.

Lung's white energy is symbolized as tiger, west, west wind, left side of body, 3-5 o'clock in the evening, autumn, sadness, longing, frost, fog, dryness, fastidious women who has craziness, strong intent, power, sadness, and kindness. To bring up white energy in our bodies, we had better eat fiery foods and strengthen our large intestine, spleen To strengthen our large intestine, we had better make our bowel movements regular and stimulate the wrist of thumb's root. I think good propolis can make white light twinkle in our bodies, too.

Genius is only one remove from insanity. Lung's white energy has the character of both genius and of insanity. Sadness and longing of lung's white energy can bring up completeness, sobriety and kindness. Sobriety, kindness can bring up wisdom and silent knowledge.

Sadness and longing can make our assemblage points (the core of consciousness) move into the more interior of our bodies than joy. Sadness and longing can strengthen our kidneys. Lung's sadness and longing can bring up the black energy of kidney. The black energy of kidney can give us silent knowledge (voice without voice, silent voice, the voice of God and instinct), patience, detachment, originality and bravery. The Man who has only strength is not a manly man. Man who has both strength and sadness (kindness) is a manly man. Like a manly man, white energy is complex. Goethe, the famous German dramatist (1749-1832) said "man who has not eaten bread together with tear is not worthy to talk with".

To bring up body-response, the fire in our abdomens and the immaterial fiber or the third attention which is shot out from our bodies, we have to have 6 kinds of energies which are black energy, blue energy, red energy, transparent energy, yellow energy, white energy. The lack of one kind of energy or the excess of one kind of energy weakens our body-responses, the fire in our abdomens, our immaterial fibers, third attention, health, instinct and ability.

If we have excessive red energy and have not moderate sad white energy, we become too joyful, too active, too ruthless, too sexy, too lewd. We can not keep ourselves cool, too. We become like plants that do not ripen but flourish. Plants need moderate frost to ripen.

White energy makes us sadden and long until we begin to try and accomplish something that is essential for us to become healthy, happy, and efficient. In such a way, white energy can teach us what to do. White energy is symbolized as frost and our later years. We are apt to feel sad very much in the autumn of our lives. We have to do something by all means to get rid of much sadness and to make ourselves satisfied. If we don't do so, we will be killed by too much sadness. Crops can not ripen in autumn if there is a heavy frost.

Sadness is strange and odd. It is useful and obstacle for us. It is like powerful drugs.

Mr. Clinton, the president of U.S.A has much white and green energy in his body, so I think he has experienced and known sadness well. I had often been outraged by my father so violently in my hometown house that the bone of my left wrist was broken.

When I was knocked down or kicked by my father in my early teens, I ran away from my hometown house, felt sad and wept somewhere for 1-2 hours. Then, I always began to feel relieved and relaxed. I could feel peculiar inner silence. I felt as if a cave had opened in my abdomen. Much energy ascended my central energy pipe. I was engulfed by white energy. I could see that my father regretted deeply to outrage me. It was the moment that body-response happened to me and my assemblage point (the core of consciousness) was moved into the interior of my body by sadness so that I could shoot out my immaterial fiber or third attention to my father and see through him from a distant different place.

Sadness, fear, deep anger against my father could move my assemblage point into the interior of my bodies than joy. I think it made my third attention work on for me in succession all day for the first time while playing baseball as a pitcher early in my teens (In those days, when I played a baseball as a pitcher in the playground of the elementary school, I could know every ball's destination and direction 3 feet in front of every batter. Before a batter swung a bat, I could know where to go about every ball correctly which I threw. It lasted for two days).

In addition, I often tried to leap up and float in the air like a ninja in my childhood. I often played as a ninja with one of my friends. I could not float in the air, but the back of my foot, my foot and my calf could feel the repulsion-power of the earth for a split second while leaping up. Feeling the repulsion-power of the earth made me funny very much and made me leap up again and again everyday. I think it could make my assemblage point move into the interior of my bodies and brought up my psychic ability, too. I think now it gave me silent knowledge (voice without voice) while playing baseball in my childhood, too. It is effective to strengthen your internal organs or attain the supernatural power that you make the back of your foot, your foot and your calf feel the repulsion-power and the gravity of the earth everyday for a few years. In such a way, the earth can give you a big present such as happy lucky feeling, solace, instinct, inspiration and power and can teach you the path to the universe or the unknown world.

Since the hot spring of white lukewarm water made me feel relieved, relaxed and began to cure the lamp of my underbelly and my frequent urination at the age of 51, I have begun to follow the comfortable response of my body to my surroundings. I have tried to feel comfortable or uncomfortable response of my body as possible before I go, eat, buy, meet, drink, listen, write or stay. If I feel a comfortable response of my body, I will go, eat, buy, meet, drink, listen, write or stay.

I went to Toronto in Canada which is at the bank of Lake Ontario 6 years ago because I felt relieved when I uttered the word "Toronto" a few times. The cool clear transparent atmosphere of Toronto made me relieved and relaxed when I visited Toronto. Furthermore, I felt relieved and relaxed while I was looking into the water of Lake Ontario. In spite of the fairly dirty water, I was not weary of looking into it. I entered into the water and watered my head. My head felt relieved and became clear. The stickiness and depression's fever of my head were erased by the water of Lake Ontario. I felt much white energy was ascending from Lake Ontario.

Just one hour before sun-set in the state of Quebec in Canada, I was engulfed by the beautiful, glossy, sweet, weak, kind, dry, noble, fierce, active, green-blue immaterial energy (the spirit). The most nectar at the top of my head was flowing down my body and made me enter into the peculiar inner silence and peculiar happiness that can not be described by words. I was burned coolly and sweetly.

My best power-spot place is in the state of Quebec in Canada. Modern astronomy says"Most of the universe is in absolute zero (-273,15 C?)". By the way, presumably, I tend to like cold places on the earth. Whenever I saw pure fresh snow or ice twinkling in the strong winter-sun when I was in elementary school, I was excited and my abdomen became warm even though the tip of my toes were numb due to the cold. I feel very sorry that my physical body can't visit Quebec more often. Only my immaterial fiber or third attention can often visit Quebec. I have 5 small power spots in Japan. At one of these small power spots in Japan, I feel very relaxed. It has the glossy, dry, sweet, noble, black, immaterial energy. My back tends to become warm, very comfortable and I can peek into the interior of the earth easily, but I can not be so burned there as in the state of Quebec in Canada.

Whenever I imagined The Caribbean Sea, I felt comfortable. Furthermore, the stiff lamp of my underbelly became fluid and soft. I could find my abdomen relaxed and pleased. I often enlarged my energy body to the size of a giant and made my energy body play in The Caribbean Sea as if it were a bath. So, I visited and swum in the Caribbean Sea 5 years ago after I attended the conference at The University of Wisconsin. Although I was looking at The Caribbean Sea practically for long hours, I did not lose interest in it.

I felt strong healthy pulse, surface tension, elasticity, and green energy in The Caribbean Sea. I felt as if it were a living thing. Whenever

I remember the feeling of The Caribbean Sea in Japan, the lamp of my underbelly and my frequent urination got well little by little.

In December 1995, I stayed Amazon in Brazil about for 3 weeks. My head felt relieved whenever I took a shower in Rio de Janeiro in Brazil in summer 1995. So, I visited Brazil again in December 1995 and went to the jungle region of Amazon.

The water of water service in Amazon region was yellow and sweet. It emitted the smell of mud and of sand. Whenever I took a shower and drank it, I felt relieved and relaxed. After I kept on drinking the water of Amazon, the smell of my excrement and of urine became the same smell as that of Amazon's water. Furthermore, I felt as if the region's earth between Rio Branco and Boca do Acre had been firing 10 feet in height. I felt as if the fire of Amazon's earth had burned the dirty sticky energy of my abdomen. The water and earth of Amazon has changed my constitution and made my character franker.

Some Brazil musics which Mr.R, my Brazilian friend selected from his radio could erase the stickiness of my body's central energy pipe. When I began to listen to these musics, I could feel that tickle happened to the top of my head and energy began to circulate between my head and my abdomen. The sound of these musics was light and heavy, weak and strong, noble and fierce, lovely and fearful, sexy and sober, sweet and ruthless, peaceful and nimble, cool and passionate. It can not be explained by the words on the earth. Its atmosphere was the same as those of the far distant universe and of the Holy Spirit.

I have been to Tyousi about 10 times since 5 years ago which is a famous fishing harbor 2 hours distant by car from my house. When I wondered if I went to Tyousi, I felt relieved. So, I went to Tyousi and ate raw fish at a cheap restaurant. Then, I felt more relieved. The lamp of my underbelly and my frequent urination got well more.

Furthermore, I have eaten or drunken the products grown at the region that I feel relieved or comfortable. So, I have kept on eating the rice of Akita prefecture in Japan, and sometimes drink vodka of Russia.

I wrote a fourth book in Japanese with the title-How to concentrate on your breath and stop it automatically 7 years ago because energy ascended from my abdomen while gathering material (in Chinese) for the book. I felt as if I had been burning while reading Chinese material, so I decided to write about it.

When I have to buy new color TV, air conditioner, refrigerator and so on, I stand in front of them and try to feel my body-response silently. When my body can feel relieved and relaxed about them, I will buy them.

When I stay at a Japanese-style hotel, I will stay at a hotel about which my body feels relieved and relaxed in front of a hotel. When my body feels relieved and relaxed in front of a hotel, most landlords' family live longer and happier. Three generations of landlord often live together happier in the hotel. As soon as I enter a hotel, I often ask the landlord or his wife "Your family live longer happily, don't you?". Then, I am always asked "That is right. Why do you know?". The hotel is at a power-spot whose energy is beautiful, dry, glossy.

A evangelist and pastor, Mr. Mahesh Chavda said in August in1999 in Japan "Since I moved from Florida, my many followers have begun to be fainted or drunken by the spirit in my church, All Nations Church in North Carolina in U.S.A. Many lights can be seen in my church, too. Many people have begun to come to our all-night Friday prayers from all over the country by sightseeing buses". I think it is because that he has rebuilt his church at a power-spot in North Carolina.

I can have confirmed big men were raised in the house at a power-spot whose energy is not dirty, sticky, feverish, cold, numb, or depressed, too. All big men have cleaned-up central energy pipes in their body. Their central energy pipes don't get stuck. All big men are not like twisty cucumbers. Their voices are uttered not from their mouths but from the central energy pipes of their bodies. When I visit a big man's house, my central energy pipe becomes less stuck and less sticky. I try to find the best power-spot in a big man's house and I sit down or stand there.

I saw my hometown house and garden in Kyoto prefecture 3 years ago because the former 3 generations of my family had been unhappy. Then, I could find that my hometown house and the garden had been taken over by black and gray dirty sticky energy that was a foot in thickness. This energy moved like a big flat snake. The Active Side of Infinity that was published in 1998 explains it as a mud shadow. I cleaned up the sky, surface and ground of my hometown house. Then, I was surprised to see beautiful white energy ascended to the sky from the window of my hometown house's ceiling.

Don Juan Matus says in the book, Tales of Power"Power always makes a cubic centimeter of chance available to a warrior. The warrior's art is to be perennially fluid in order to pluck it"

Useful power, devil, dirty energy body of other, or floating dirty sticky cloud sticks a pipe into our physical bodies or energy bodies while we are dreaming at night or moving in the daytime. We have to pluck or enter a pipe of useful power which is beautiful, dry, glossy, cool, active, of abandon, of largesse, and of humor. I have begun to find the hole of such a pipe's tip in the sky while dreaming since 3 years ago. My energy body has approached it and entered into it while dreaming. After going through such a pipe, there exist beautiful another world which is 2-4 km in diameter.

A third time my energy body tried to go through such a pipe 3 years ago, it was broken. Suddenly something like an exhausted snake ran away from my central energy pipe. Furthermore, something like 20-30 tenacious strong black army ants ran away from the lamp of my underbelly. Since then, the lamp of my underbelly, my frequent urination and the trouble of my spine have been cured. They had been torturing me for 25 years since a massager woman injured my spine at the age of 31.

In spite of the complete recovery, I have been so careful that I have still kept on taking an hour stroll and practicing the reverse movement of my body everyday in order to strengthen the muscle of the back and of my abdomen. It has prevented the bone of my spine from turning aside.

There have been hundreds of body exercises, yoga, meditation, prays, mantra, stares, breath's way, fasting. Many practices are written in Carlos Castaneda's books, too. If we test for 2-3 months per way, we can not finish testing the ways of all practices by we pass away. I have begun to practice them since the age of 37. Especially from age of 45 until the age of 51, I had been practicing them for 7-8 hours everyday. Then, at last I felt as if I had been imprisoned and felt sad.

Buddha had been practicing many ways involving fasting crazily for 6 years 2500 years ago and stopped practicing them at the age of 35. He taught his followers (1)the origin of pain and of depression is not following comfortable body's response (2)don't do what your body feel uncomfortable (3)what your body feel comfortable is accurate (4)do what your body feel comfortable and your pain and depression will be eliminated

At present Mr. Eugene T Gendlin teaches the same way in the book with the title-Focusing. Mr.James Redfield and Carol Adrienne introduce the same way in the book with the title-The Celestine Prophecy, too.

I had cured the lamp of my underbelly, my frequent urination and the trouble of my spine by the grace of following my body's responses. Whenever I glanced at the mountain near Karuizawa through a window of a train, my head felt relieved and relaxed. That is to say, my body tried to teach me what to do to cure the lamp of my underbelly, my frequent urination and the trouble of my spine as the above mentioned sentence.

If I had been stupid or donkey enough to ignore such a body's response to the end, I might have died of bladder cancer already.

Don Juan Matus taught such body responses to his disciple, he late Mr.Carlos Castaneda (1)tickle happens at the top of head and descends to the back, waist, and womb (in such a case, assemblage point (the core of consciousness) moves into the interior of the body and we can feel accurate decision making or judgment without an illusion) (2)see the subtle third attention or the spirit (3)see the immaterial fiber of the universe (4)sound happens in the recess of throat as if a wooden pipe were snapped (5)feel as if a cave opened in the abdomen and energy ascends from the abdomen (6)overwhelming premonition (7)can hear the voice without voice on the back of ear(8)feel as if we could perceive about two places or exist at two places simultaneously.

Don Juan Matus says that in these cases we can shoot out the immaterial fibers or our subtle third attention to an object from our bodies, can judge it accurately and control it. In such a case, what we imagine will be realized soon.

Mr. Eugene T Gendlin introduces body-responses in his book with the title-Focusing (1)we begin to feel relieved and relaxed (2)begin to take a deep breath (3)stiff abdomen turns to be fluid and relaxed. Mr. James Redfield and Carol Adrienne introduce body-response in their book with the title-The Celestine Prophecy "we feel beautiful, relieved or relaxed when we see or visit someone, something, some place that can give us something useful".

Some executive says in the book with the title-Executive ESP "When I have made an accurate decision, I feel a click".

By constricting anus 100 times in succession and denting navel 100 times in succession everyday following the life style of the long-lived British, we have to develop the muscles of abdomen, waist, hip and thigh firmly. To bring up or strengthen our body-responses, our immaterial fibers and our third attention and cure or prevent depression, we had better constrict anus 100 times in succession and dent navel 100 times in succession everyday, burn the fire from within our bodies and develop the muscles of abdomen, waist, hip and thigh firmly. We have to be able to petrify the muscle of abdomen like steel and soften it like water intentionally. Needless to say, good complexion and rejuvenation (grow at least 10-20 years younger) have to happen to us, too. Somehow, staring at something and concentrating on it for more than one hour everyday can erase the bad stickiness of our bodies, rotate the vortexes of our bodies, burn the fire from within our bodies, shoot out our immaterial fibers or third attention from our bodies, succeed in concentrating on and develop the muscles of abdomen, waist, hip and thigh firmly, too.

I can guess that don Juan Matus and don Genaro had developed the muscles of abdomen, waist, hip, thigh firmly more than don Juan Matus' teacher. Julian Osario. So, they are more powerful, can see through more than Julian Osario. I have not sufficiently developed these muscles firmly because I had been tortured for long years by the trouble of my spine, the lamp of my underbelly and my frequent urination. It is my weak point that I will have to overcome by all means.

Poor or flabby abdomen, waist, hip and thigh have much dirty stickiness, can not rotate vortexes of body, can not burn the fire from within body, can not give us happy lucky feeling, can shoot out neither immaterial fiber nor the third attention from body, can not make us concentrate on anything, can not give us supernatural power, can not make us realize what we imagine and can not make the body-response happen to the surroundings.

The late Mr. Mihara, the famous baseball manager in Japan had fired the baseball player who had lost the muscles of his hip and of his waist. Whenever Mr. Mihara wondered if some player of his team was fired, he entered a public bath with the player and peeped at the muscles of the player's hip and of the player's waist.

In this respect, most of us, most pastors and most psychic teachers are apt to have the bad muscles (poor, flabby, fat or stiff) of abdomen, waist, hip, thigh because most of us and they are apt to go anywhere not on foot but by car. Most of us and they are apt to do no body-exercise at all and eat too much, too. Needless to say, women have to strengthen her wombs. Constricting anus 100 times and denting navel 100 times everyday can strengthen womb, too.

I think Christ and Buddha did not teach "we have to make a point of body exercise or sports to cure or prevent depression and become healthy-happy-efficient" to us 2000-2500 years ago. I think it is right because people in those days had to walk and work without cars or machines. They moved their bodies well everyday and did not need more stroll, body-exercise, or sports than at present. To the contrary, at present most of us, most pastors and most psychic teachers are apt to need more stroll, body-exercise or sports everyday than long years ago because of cars, machines or too much eating.

Only praying, reading doctrines, singing, meditation and worrying about management everyday are apt to weaken their bodies and hearts easily. I think most pastors and most psychic teachers are apt not to make the fire burn within their bodies, too. To survive and prosper at present, Christianity and Buddhism had better change their doctrines according to the change of our society.

Constricting anus 100 times and denting navel 100 times everyday following the life style of long-lived British and doing 3-week fasting can be compared to(1) shadowboxing(2)or a maintenance garage for broken fighters.

If we only respect constricting anus 100 times and denting navel 100 times everyday following the life style of long-lived British and respect doing 3-week fasting, and ignore following comfortable body-responses, we will be compared to (1)prizefighters avoiding any fight (2)or fighters abandoned in a maintenance garage although their radars and guided missiles have been repaired.

If we only respect following our body-response, ignore constricting anus 100 times and denting navel 100 times everyday following the life style of long-lived British and ignore doing 3-week fasting, we will be compared to (1)prizefighters hating training (2)or fighters flying without repairing their broken radars and guided missiles.

We can not become strong prizefighters without long hard training. On the contrary, if we practice only training and avoid any fight, we will become timid and become like a rotten apple. If we fight and are beaten, we only study why to be beaten and strengthen ourselves through training. If we are so proud of our strength as to hate training after we become strong prizefighters, we will be beaten deadly sooner or later. So, I think we had better respect both doing some proper body-exercise (for example, constricting anus 100 times-denting navel 100 times) every-day following the life style of long-lived British-doing 3-week fasting and following comfortable body-response.

Precisely, above-mentioned body-responses have not happened to most of us at all. Furthermore, most of us ignore them because of no good reason to believe if body-responses happen to them by any chance. Complaints (about health, opposite sex, son, daughter, parents, work, boss, money or post), dirty energy bodies of others and devils have given most of us much stickiness, depression's fever, coldness or numbness. This much stickiness, depression's fever, coldness or numb-ness has broken the direction signals of our bodies. So, body-response has not worked on for us.

Furthermore, we have not been taught to respect or follow body-responses in schools or companies. We have been taught to ignore them there. We have been taught to respect and follow plausible reasons. For example, we have been taught to believe in the prospects of stock prices that have plausible reasons. Most of us ignore body-responses if they happen to most of us.

In most cases, to repair the direction signals of our bodies and make body-responses work on for us, we had better do some proper body-exercise (for example, constricting anus 100 times and denting navel 100 times) everyday following the life style of long-lived British and do 3-week fasting. After good complexion, rejuvenation, good appetite, good sleeping, good bowel movement, soft shoulder, happy feeling, subtle breath, dryness, and gloss begin to happen to us little by little, body-responses are apt to happen to us little by little. That is to say, body-responses will happen to us little by little after we begin to develop the muscles of abdomen, waist, hip, thigh firmly, begin to get rid of poor, flabby, fat, or stiff abdomen-waist-hip-thigh, begin to rotate the vortexes of our bodies, begin to burn the fire from within our bodies, begin to erase the much dirty stickiness of our bodies and begin to have good complexion by constricting anus 100 times and denting navel 100 times everyday following the life style of long-lived British and by doing 3-week fasting.

If body-responses begin to happen to us, we had better run a risk to follow them at our perils. If we are so timid that we can not follow them, we had better follow the body-response to our hobbies, eating, furniture and something that don't need much money. At least, we can respect and follow the body-responses to our private lives as much as possible.

Successful founders in various channels, enterprisers, pioneers, skilled craftsmen and masters are apt to ignore plausible reasons, respect their body-responses and venture to follow their body-responses. They are often uneducated people. They have not been poisoned by education. So, we had better make friends with them to imitate such features.

First of all, you had better test your body-response to my book with the help of your body-response. How about your body-response to my book just before you begin to read it? The scripture says "like a baby, you had better thirst for the voice of God". The voice of God is one of the body-responses. It is a voice without voice on the back of your ear. Can you hear such a voice about my book just before you begin to read my book? Does the voice without voice (silent voice, silent knowledge and the ascent of your kidney's black energy) ascend from your abdomen to the back of your left ear?. Or, can your body feel comfortable or uncomfortable about my book just before you begin to read it or while reading it? Can your body feel the color, smell, touch's sense, sound or flavor of my book?

This is the example of my reader's body-response to my contribution to the newsgroup of depression.

Subject:   Re: How to good-by depression 12
From:      Aah
Date:      Thu, 13 January 2000 10:57 AM EST
Message-id:
Newsgroup: depression
In article, Hiroyuki

Nishigaki writes

    3 week fasting can make you excrete a bucketful of old black
excrement(4-5 kg) and make your bowel movement regular.
Why does this make me feel better about my tooth?

    ——

    Aah~~~~~~~~~~~~~~~~~~~~~~~~~~~~~~~~~~~~~~~~~~~~~~~
~~~~~~~~~~~~~~~~~~~~~~~~~~~~~~~~

    The opinions given above may be mine. They might also
ust be what I feel like saying right now, okay?

   Please, estimate my book not by plausible reasons but by your
body-response. Goethe .the famous German dramatist said "we are
tricked not by body-responses but by reason". If no body-response
happens to you at all, you had better realize that your body-response
has been broken. So, you had better enter a training gym, or maintenance garage for a while (at least for 3 years).

   In most cases, if you remember your life in detail at least 50 times,
you will realize that you have tried to do new many things and chase
men or women one after another ignoring your body-response or not
waiting body-response and failed one after another. So, don Juan
Matus says "It is dangerous and vain for us to act before body-
response happens to us".

# Part 7 Check your condition

When we burn the fire from within our bodies, erase the stickiness of our bodies, have good complexion, neither get stuck nor depressed and have good body-response, our assemblage points (the core of consciousness) can move into the interior of our bodies and our immaterial fibers ( or the third attention ) can shoots out to an outside object from our bodies and succeed in concentrate on it. Then, we can accomplish something. In such a case, we are neither proud nor careless. We are not in illusion but in reality. That is to say, we can say that we have dependable good self-importance, self-image and trust. To accomplish something, we had better check whether or not we have dependable good self-importance, self-image and trust.

I think it is effective to cure or prevent depression and become happy-healthy-efficient that you had better often check whether or not (1)you eat in moderation (2)have good complexion (3)make friends with danger or death(4)have good self-importance (5) have dependable trust (6)have good repentance (7) burn the fire from within your body and clean up the central energy pipe of your body (8)walk in the right way (9)say thank you, too. I intend to explain them by turns.

The Second Ring of Power by the late Mr. Carlos Castaneda says "A warrior eats quietly, and slowly, and very little at a time. Don Juan Matus told her (La Gorda) that a warrior eats four mouthfuls of food at one time. A while later he eats another four mouthfuls and so on. A warrior also walks miles and miles everyday. Her eating weakness never let her walk. She broke it by eating four mouthfuls every time and by walking. Sometimes, she walked all day and all night. That was the way she lost the fat on her buttocks. But, stalking your weakness is not enough to drop them. She said you can stalk them from now to dooms-day and it won't make a bit of difference. What a warrior really needs in order to be an impeccable stalker is to have a purpose. The warrior's purpose is to enter into the other world (the universe, the spirit)"

I think we can neither become happy-healthy-efficient nor prevent-cure depression unless we eat in moderation. Yoga book says "However we endeavor, we can not succeed in accomplishing the purpose of yoga unless we eat in moderation". The purpose of yoga is to be able to shoot out our immaterial fibers (which is called Samyama in yoga world) or third attention (which is called Purusha in yoga world) to an object from our bodies, judge it, and control it. That is to say, it is the success of concentration. The last purpose of yoga is to be able to recognize our third attention like a smoke in a treasure-chest, handle it, and catch on the spirits.

Ancient Buddhist priests ate once a day by noon. When I visited most their remains in India about 20 years ago, I thought they walked for 5-6 hours everyday to gather foods around other ordinary people's houses. After enough walk, they sat and meditated everyday. Owing to enough walks, long sitting and meditation could not weaken their bodies or hearts. To the contrary, most of us are apt to go anywhere by car and eat too much. Furthermore, most pastors and psychic teachers are apt to pray, read doctrines, sing, meditate and worry about management (money?) everyday without enough walks or body-exercise. So, our physical bodies and their physical bodies are apt to be weakened by the lack of enough walks and of body exercise and by eating too much.

I am apt to eat too much and quickly. I have tried to finish eating before sunset, but failed in doing so. I weigh 10 kilograms over the standard weight. Whenever I eat dinner too much after sunset, I can neither shoot out my immaterial fiber or third attention to an outside object from my body nor change my dream easily. In such a case, I can not concentrate my immaterial fiber or third attention on anything at all. The ability to imagine happy good feeling and the ability of supernatural power decline, too. I am confined to dirty stickiness, the fever of depression, coldness, or numbness like heavy oil sea, sludge or sewage. I am confined to irritation, self-pity, foolishness, indecision, depression and timidity that are the core of unhappy-unhealthy-inefficient individual and home. Next day, it is fairly difficult for me to shoot out my immaterial fiber or third attention from my body. I am still fairly like a blockhead.

I am so foolish that I have failed in eating in moderation and losing my weight since 10 years ago. Although I have understood the obstacle of eating too much and of fatness, I have failed. So, since 4 years ago I have decided not to order new business suits before I succeed in losing my weight by 10 kilograms. Now, there have remained 2-3 proper winter business suites. I have been in deadly earnest to try to lose my weight since 20 days ago.

I have tried to eat four mouthfuls of food at one time in the morning. I have tried to chew a mouthful of food 100 times. I have tried to eat so at one time in the afternoon. I have eaten so twice a day since 20 days ago so that I have lost my weight by 5 kilograms. I will have to lose my weight by more 5 kilograms.

I have done 3 week-fasting 6 times since 20 years ago. When I finished 3-week fasting, I lost my weight by 8-10 kilograms. I excreted a bucketful of old black excrement (4-5 kilograms), so I lost my weight precisely by 4-5 kilograms. After fasting, everything becomes delicious. I have good appetite so that I am apt to eat too much and gain weight again.

When I concentrate on my breath almost all day during fasting, I can feel that stickiness, the fever of depression, coldness and numbness in my body begin to resolve and exhaust from my shoulder like a dirty gray smoke. I can feel that fasting can discharge bad unnecessary energy from my body and purify my body. It is such a bad unnecessary energy that makes our immaterial fibers or third attention (the core of consciousness) shut into our bodies like a bird in heavy oil sea and makes us like a blockhead. Devils and dirty energies of others like such a bad unnecessary energy and stick to us like vultures, hyenas or maggots if we have such a bad unnecessary energy. When I cure a patient or teach someone, I feel I am often attacked by the devil that has stuck to a patient or someone.

Mr. Nanboku Mizuno (1756-1834), the most famous Japanese man of physiognomy said "Good luck is dependent on eating in moderation. However good physiognomy (look) you have, misfortune will happen to you sooner or later as long as you eat too much or are a epicure. However bad physiognomy you have, considerable or moderate luck will happen to you as long as you eat in moderation or are not an epicure".

He was out of a gangster. To study physiognomy, he worked for a barber, public bath and crematory. He studies as far as many sex organs and anuses.

The more he studied physiognomy, the more mistakes he made in physiognomy. Some day, he guessed that eating in moderation and not-being an epicure are the most important points of physiognomy. Since then, he asked "Are you apt to eat too much or are you a epicure?" before he predicted someone's luck. As a result, he could hit the mark ten times out of ten about predicting many people's future lucks. So, he could become so famous for physiognomy that he had more than 1000 disciples in Japan about 200 years ago.

In addition, he thought that the second most important point of physiognomy next to eating in moderation is beautiful glossy color of red, of yellow, and of white on the surface of face. He said "pale blue, pale white, dirty black red, dirty yellow, not-glossy red, not-glossy yellow, not-glossy white and not-glossy black on the surface of face are the omens of misfortune. Beautiful glossy color of red, of yellow, and of white on the surface of face is the omen of good luck". If your internal organ weakens, dirty not-glossy color will happen to the part of your face's surface where there is the gate or entrance of energy channel connected with your internal organ.

When good complexion happens to you, good bowel movement, good sleeping, soft shoulder, good sex, subtle breath, rejuvenation (grow at least 10-20 years younger) happen to you, too. As a result, you do not feel stuck or depressed, can get rid of poor, flabby, fat, or stiff abdomen-waist-hip-thigh, enjoy happy good feeling. In such a case, the color of your dream is not dirty dark color but a beautiful lively color.

You are suffering from misfortune as long as the color of your dream is dirty dark, pale, dirty black red, dirty brown, not-glossy, or not-lively. When you can enjoy a beautiful glossy lively dream, good luck happens to you. When you begin to eat in moderation or do fasting, you will be able to begin to dream a beautiful glossy lively dream.

Mr. Nanboku Mizuno, the famous man of physiognomy said "The origin of poverty, downfall, disease, discord (over wife, husband, son, daughter, junior partner, associate, fellow worker or boss), sterility, divorce, juvenile delinquent, accident or dying young is eating too much or being a epicure. The misfortune's origin of son or of daughter is parent's eating too much or parent's being a epicure. Those who are suffering from such a misfortune had better eat in moderation or stop being an epicure and can emerge from such a misfortune. That is the most important secret of my physiognomy".

My acquaintance could not become a prime minister of Japan and died of cancer several years ago. Owing to his attribute which were the same as those of a warrior such as abandon, largess, humor, ruthlessness, cunnings, patience, sweet and making friends with danger or death, he started from scratch and rose to No 2 in the Japan political world. He had keen scent, ran the risk of losing whatever he possessed after careful calculation and could shoot out his immaterial fiber or third attention to an object from his body. I can remember that he often emitted his third attention from his body about 25 years ago. He had often burned from within his abdomen. I had liked him because he had many same attribute as those of a warrior which were explained by don Juan Matus. He had taught me about them involuntarily for about 25 years. I owe him much gratitude.

Some day, he asked me in secret "Do you think I will be able to become a prime minister?". I replied to him "If you keep on being healthy, you will surely become a prime minister sooner or later. But, I think it matters little if you can become a prime minister or not. You had better do any good act for Japan or the world that is thought of by you as if you were a prime minister. Now that you have become one of the bosses and have big influence over the Japan political world, you can do so from now on. As long as you do so, you never become mortified if you can not become a Prime Minister. Without the post of a Prime Minister, you can do the same work as that of a Prime Minister if you want". He was much pleased to hear my thought. He said to me "Good advice. You can really have begun to talk good thing, can't you?".

After all, the big man of the Japan political world died of cancer not becoming a Prime Minister of Japan. I think it was because that he ate too much, was fat and began to have bad complexion little by little. His wife said to me "I have often said to my husband that? For your health, you had better live in moderation?. But, he never follows my advice. I have given up".

Kennedy Junior (the son of the former U.S.A president) died in his own airplane crash over the Pacific in summer in 1999. I wonder if he had eaten too much or been an epicure? Furthermore, I wonder if he had bad complexion?

In this respect, you can judge soundly what you do with the help of your complexion. Whatever you do is proper as long as your complexion becomes better so that you can grow younger.

Don Juan Matus says in the book with the title-The Teaching of Don Juan "Anything is one of a million paths. If a warrior feels that he should not follow it, he must not stay with it under any condition. He must look at every path closely and deliberately. There is a question that a warrior has to ask, mandatory: Does this path have a heart? A path without a heart is never enjoyable. On the other hand, a path with heart is easy-it does not make a warrior work at linking it; it makes for a joyful journey; as long as a man follows it, he is one with it". You can transpose the word "heart" to the word "good complexion" in the above-mentioned sentence.

By the way, Nanboku Mizuno?the famous man of physiognomy said "Those who live near the river flowing down to the east are apt to become unhappy or unhealthy". Somehow, I feel much irritated and tired while moving to the west on foot or by car near the river flowing down to the east. I feel as if I were pulled to the east by some energy. I have heard that those who keep on working or sitting for long hours everyday pointing the east have become so irritated, tired and dull that they have suffered from neurosis or become insane or an alcoholic at last. I think you had better often change your aspect everyday not to become irritated and tired.

There are two kinds of self-importance. A good self-importance is to imagine happy good feeling, positive thinking, or positive self-image and make it realize because we can shoot out our immaterial fibers or our third attention from our bodies to an object, judge and control it. Just before it is realized, a body-response will happen to us. Such a body-response is as followers-(1)a tickle happens at the top of head and descends to the back, waist, and womb(in such a case, assemblage point moves into the interior of the body and we can feel accurate decision making or judgment without an illusion) (2)see the subtle third attention or the spirit (3)see the immaterial fiber of the universe(4)sound happens in the recess of throat as if a wooden pipe were snapped (5)feel as if a cave opened in the abdomen and energy ascends from the abdomen (6)overwhelming premonition (7)can hear a voice without voice on the back of ear (8)feel as if we could perceive about two places or exist at two places simultaneously (9) begin to feel relieved and relaxed (10)begin to take a deep breath (11)stiff abdomen turns to be fluid and relaxed (12) feel beautiful (13) feel a click.

Only when we can burn the fire from within our bodies and erase our bad stickiness with the help of the fire so that good complexion, good sleeping, good appetite, good bowel movement, good sex, soft shoulder, rejuvenation, subtle breath happen to us, such a body-response happen to us and we can shoot out our immaterial fibers or third attention to an outside object from our bodies so that we can concentrate on it and have a good self-importance. In such a case, our assemblage points (the core of consciousness) move to the point of undoubt so that we can trust our happy good feelings, positive thinking, or positive self-image.

To the contrary, a rotten self-importance is to imagine happy good feeling, positive thinking, or positive self-image and not to be able to make it realize because we can not burn the fire from within our bodies, can not erase our bad stickiness with the help of fire, can not shoot out our immaterial fibers or our third attention to an object from our bodies, can not judge it accurately, can not control it, and can not concentrate on it.

In such a case, body-response will never happen to us while imaging. Our bad stickiness, bad complexion, bad sleeping, bad appetite, bad bowel movement, bad sex, stiff shoulder, growing older, rough breath and depression make our immaterial fiber or third attention confined to our bodies so that we have a rotten self-importance. Then, our assemblage points can not move into the interior of our bodies. If we trust false happy good feelings, false positive thinking, or false positive self-image, we will be proud, conceited, arrogant, blowers. Big men, founders, pioneers or enterprisers always have rotten self-importance since 3-5 years earlier before they are disgraced. Then, they become proud, conceited, arrogant, blowers ignoring body-response or not waiting body-response.

If we keep on having rotten self-importance and fail in realizing happy good feeling, positive thinking, or positive self-image in succession, we will begin to keep on indulging in self-pity.

Buddha said in India 2500 years ago "We had better check whether or not we can trust what we imagine, think, or plan. We have to learn how to trust or what to trust as possible". Don Juan Matus says "What we need to do to allow magic to get hold of us is to banish doubts from our minds. Once doubts are banished, anything is possible"(Power of Silence).

I think we can practice Tensegrity more merrily than other body exercise. Tensegrity can balance our energy and make our awareness keen. But, I think it is fairly difficult for us to make the fire burn from within and to clean up our central energy pipes of our bodies with the help of Tensegrity.

The homepage of infoseek (abcnews.go.com) says that The Associated Press LOSANGELS reported on June in 1998 Mr. Carlos Castaneda died of liver cancer on April 27 in 1998. He was believed to be 72. The Los Angeles Times reported that he was cremated immediately and his ashes were spirited away to Mexico. The relationship with his daughter, opposite sexes and his parents or the guilt about his childhood friend who was injured by him seemed to have deprived Mr. Carlos Castaneda of light spring breeze's feeling and joy. If we lose such a happy good feeling, liver and heart will weaken. As a result, I think we will have bad complexion, get stuck and depressed, and have to die of cancer, heart disease or high blood pressure sooner or later at last.

If we can make the fire burn from within and to clean up our central energy pipes, we can recover the good feeling of light spring breeze, of joy and of bravery, can strengthen liver, heart and kidney and can cure or prevent depression. Good complexion, rejuvenation, good bowel movement, good sleeping, good appetite, good sex and subtle breath can happen to us. Furthermore, we can easily thank someone, some beautiful scene, some food, the earth and so on so that we can recover from such a disease. It is the energy of our central energy pipes that is so-called inner-God or Phenix or the strongest third attention.

I think (1)constricting anus 100 times in succession, denting navel 100 times in succession and doing bowel movement 6 times everyday (2) 3 week-fasting (3) concentrating your breath almost all day for 3 weeks (4)tempering your energy by the way of Chinese style(5)beckoning the spirits (6) following your body-response are the most effective to make the fire burn from within and to clean up your central energy pipe of your body.

Next to the most effective ways are as follows. (7)repenting yourself (8)making your head pay attention to the universe, your abdomen pay attention to the inner space, and your feet pay attention to the interior of the earth simultaneously as often as possible whenever you are free (9)concentrating your attention on your central energy pipe and clean up it everyday(10)drinking 1,8 liter warm water with a little salt just before sun-rise everyday and vomit it from the stomach(don't do so if you are suffering from high blood pressure, heart disease, or heavy stomach ulcer) for 2 weeks once a year.

(11)the right way of walking-"The warrior, first by curling his finger, drew attention to the arms; and then by looking, without focusing your eye, at any point directly in front of you on the arc that started at the tip of your feet and ended above the horizon, you literally flooded your tonal(the right side of your body, the first attention)with information. The tonal became silent"(Tale of Power)(12)staring at something with eyebrows stretched, shoot out your immaterial fiber or third attention to an outside object from your body and succeeding in concentrating on it (13)seeing or making friends with happy-healthy-efficient people, big men, founders, pioneers and enterprisers or listening to their voices as long as they have good self-importance(14)finding the best power-spot and stay there(15)talking, seeing or acting with abandon, largess and humor-are effective for you to burn the fire from within your body and clean up their central energy pipes, too. Needless to say, this fire can burn the bad stickiness of your body that has confined your immaterial fiber or third attention to your body and has made it useless or dead.

If you often repent yourself easily, such repenting yourself is little effective. If you have been devious and stubborn very much for long years, recognizing your stupidity and repenting yourself are one of the most effective. In such a case, your assemblage point (the core of consciousness) will be able to move into the interior of your body. The spirit may descend to you for the first time, help you and give you supernatural power. When don Juan Matus recognized his stupidity, said thank you to his teacher, accepted his death and repented himself deeply for the first time, he could make the fire burn from within and clean up his central energy pipe. Then, He fused himself to the emanations of the black energy (which is called Eagle in Carlos Castaneda's books) at large, and glided into infinity (black energy) for the first time. I think it seemed to be the biggest memorial to him. In this respect, Mr. Carlos Castaneda seemed to get so perverse that he could not have repented himself as deeply as his teacher, don Juan Matus did. This may be another origin for Mr.Carlos Castaneda not to become a successor to don Juan Matus.

Repentance is like a powerful drug that is both medicine and poison for us. When you repent yourself and recognize your stupidity, you will have a body-response such as (1) feeling as if a cave opened in the abdomen and energy ascends from the abdomen (it is the evidence that the fire begins to burn from within and your central energy pipe begins to be cleaned up) (2) beginning to take a deep breath (3) stiff abdomen's turning to be fluid and relaxed. In such a case, good repentance has happened to you and your assemblage point has moved into the interior of your body so that you can shoot out your immaterial fiber or third attention to an outside object from your body, judge and control it. You can begin to judge an outside object accurately or realize what you imagine or recover from disease or become healthier or feel happier. Good repentance can strengthen your physical body and energy body. Such a good repentance is medicine.

To the contrary, you will not have such a body-response such as (1)(2)(3) when you repent yourself and recognize your stupidity. In such a case, bad repentance has happened to you and your assemblage point has not moved into the interior of your body so that you can neither shoot out your immaterial fiber or third attention to an object from your body nor judge-control it. Such a bad repentance is called self-pity. You can not begin to judge accurately or can not realize what you imagine or can not recover from disease or can not become healthy or can not feel happier. Bad repentance called self-pity can weaken your physical body and energy body further. Such a bad repentance is a poison.

Good repentance is apt to happen to you when you can recognize your stupidity calmly, lively, concretely and minutely at your power-spot. Furthermore, it will happen to you easily when good complexion, rejuvenation, good bowel movement, good appetite, moderation of eating, good sleeping, good sex, soft shoulder, and subtle breath begin to happen to you little by little. If you can not repent yourself under such a condition, you are compared to the bird that falls into heavy oil sea and flounders desperately. It is bad repentance called self-pity. Unhappy-unhealthy-inefficient people are apt to do bad repentance called self-pity.

We have to become modest enough to wonder if our self-importance, trust and repentance are dependable. But, usual much modesty is apt to hate danger, death or hell so that it avoids adventure, risk and desperate action. Usual much modesty is poison, so it weakens our physical bodies and energy bodies. When we become well timed and make a dash at danger, death or hell following the tactics made by your body-response, we can often break through it. At that time, our immaterial fiber or third attention confined to our bodies can be shot out from our bodies and can judge-control danger, death or hell accurately. In such a case, danger, death, or hell often runs away from us. Big men, founders, pioneers and enterprisers are good at this way. Whenever I go skiing, I ski on the most dangerous place without a stop.

Don Juan Matus could not swim. His teacher, nagual Julian Osario threw him into the flood. When he accepted his death in the flood, he could calm down and enter into the peculiar inner silence. Then, his energy body was shot out of his physical body for the first time and could approach the riverbank. I think it was the second biggest memorial to him.

I was on the brink of being killed by injection by Japanese at the age of 6 in China. I have often remembered this scene. At that time, I did not fear at all, relaxed, calmed down and behaved naturally. I think behaving in such a manner made my immaterial fiber or third attention work on for me and saved my life. I slipped out a few minutes before injection. About 100 Japanese children standing around me were killed by injection. When Japanese repatriated from the northeastern region of China after the defeat of world war 2, Japanese often killed their children in China because their children were a drag on their coming back to Japan safely.

The Wheel of times says "His teacher, Julian Osario was a tubercular man who was never cured, but who lived to be perhaps 107 years old ( on the earth), always walking along the edge of the abyss. Walking on the edge of the abyss meant the battle of a warrior enhanced to such a degree that every second counted. On the single moment of weakness would have thrown nagual Julian Osario into that abyss".

In this respect, Mr. Carlos Castaneda did not seem to make friends with danger or death. I think it seemed to be one of the origins for him to be unable to become a successor to don Juan Matus, too.

I like nagual Julian Osalio because he always walked along the edge of the abyss. I often imagine that I walk along the edge of the abyss in Mexico as if I were Julian Osario. I respect him because he kept on having the power to explode the energetic core of his abdomen in his central energy pipe until the age of 107 on the earth in spite of his disease, could explode it and could fuse with the universe at last without losing his consciousness.

While walking in the right way of walking, the sky just above the horizon seems like a female womb or the secret door of another world or the body of opposite sex. Then, you can enter into or touch it. It seems like a rope ladder that a helicopter hangs, too. If your immaterial fiber or third attention can catch it, your immaterial fiber or third attention will be lifted to the universe. It seems like a bending intent of the earth, too. You can catch it, make it straight upward and make it shoot out to the universe from the earth.

Furthermore, the sky just above the horizon can erase your stickiness and temper your energy body. While keeping on walking in such way for 3-4 hours without rest or soft drink, I seldom become tired. I think the right way of walking can make you healthier and stronger. It seems to multiply the ability for you to move in your dream and to change your dream freely. There are many kinds of devils such as a mud shadow in the inner space or on the surface of earth whose size is half an inch-the same size of France. They live anywhere. They are apt to stick to sleeping human being and absorb the energy of human being. When I notice them and get angry or trample under foot, they are apt to run away. I think the right way of walking can multiply the ability to shut out such devils from your body.

I often make the energy of my hand and of my elbow catch or break through the sky just above the horizon. This is a good way to make hand and elbow sensitive.

I feel don Juan Matus and don Genaro ate four mouthfuls of food at one time and walked miles and miles everyday on the earth. They seemed to eat in more moderation and walked more than Mr. Carlos Castaneda and me. So, I can see their legs and waists of their energy bodies are much stronger than those of Mr. Carlos Castaneda and me. I have taken for a walk for an hour everyday since 20 years ago and have walked for 3-4 hours once a week or once a month since 10 years ago. I am 59 year old Japanese and have grown 10-20 years old younger. But, don Juan Matus looked younger on the earth than his son who was a career soldier in his mid-sixties. Growing at least 10-20 years old younger is the evidence to make the fire burn from within.

I think that eating so and walking so everyday can make you feel happier, make the fire burn from within your abdomen, cure or prevent depression and can make you grow much younger. I think you will never die of cancer as long as you do so at least a few times a week. I think it is a good weapon to fight against the last enemy called Old Age. I owe much gratitude to Mr.Carlos Castaneda because he was taught about it by don Juan Matus and taught it to me through his books.

There are hundreds of ways to temper our bodies and energy bodies. If we begin to know many ways, we are apt to rove from one way to another, skip and end up practicing no way. So, those who know many ways are apt to die of cancer, of heart disease or of high blood pressure or be unable to live long. The teacher who teaches how to temper physical body and energy body are apt to have the same inclination. Knowing is not practicing. I am careful not to become so because I know many ways. Only knowing eating four mouthfuls of food at one time and walking in the right way everyday for long years is much effective for us than knowing many ways, skipping and ending up practicing no way.

I have read about 2000 books about psychic world, religion, body exercise and another world for 30 years. But, most books have been useless for me after all. I think I have wasted time on reading many books and it has weakened my physical body and energy body fairly.

I can have noticed one of the devils which has stuck to me or stolen into me or been floating above me. It is the devil that has prodded me to do something hurriedly or has made me endeavor to do something busily or has made me trapped in somewhere. This devil has made me a mouse in a rotating ring. This devil seems to have has made me read many books, too. This devil has made me a slavery of book. In such a case, good body-response has never happened to me and I feel gloomy and depressing. Then, my immaterial fiber or third attention is confined to my body and can not work on for me because good body-response has never happened to me. As a result, this devil has made me have undependable self-importance, undependable trust and self-pity. This devil has made my eyes severe or sticky or irritated or restless. I am confined to an illusion. I can not realize what I imagine or think of. You have been stolen into by the same type of devil as that of my devil, haven't you?

For me, this devil seems as if it were tenacious sticky snake whose color is transparent and gray because it has lived in my bones and my body for about 40 years. I have begun to fight against it since a year ago. I have tried to make more beautiful stronger different fire burn from within my body strengthening the function of my radiator (white energy of my lung). I will burn this devil if this devil has kept on staying and interfered in me. In these days, I buy and read a book only when I can feel good body-response (for example, I can feel relieved or relaxed or light) glancing at a book without opening a book in a bookstore. Furthermore, I have tried to change my eyes for better when I can notice I have bad eyes again. It is because we can not beckon the spirit as long as we have bad eyes. Bad eyes can beckon not the spirit but devils. Bad eyes can beckon not good opposite sex but bad opposite sex, too. Good eyes that have the feeling of abandon, largesse, humor can beckon the spirit and good opposite sexes.

So, instead of reading many books, you had better do some proper body-exercise following the life style of long-lived British, concentrate on your breath almost all day for 3 weeks at a power-spot to stop your breath automatically, talk, see and act with abandon, largess and humor to shoot out your immaterial fiber or third attention and concentrate on it, do fasting, run the risk at your peril and walk in the right way. They will teach you more than reading many books.

In most cases, a bad feeling such as that of a ruthless, shameless, crass mercenary, and of a super-sensitive, tormented artist is brought about by the devil that has the same bad feelings. Such a devil sticks to or steals into someone so that it brings about the same bad feeling to someone and tortures-weakens someone. I felt I had become fairly timid since 3 years ago, so that a year ago I could find the black brown timid devil had stolen into and lived in my body. If you can notice new different bad feeling, you had better check your body and shut out the devil which has the same bad feeling from your body.

You had better study the difference between the voice of unhealthy-unhappy-inefficient people and the voice of healthy-happy-efficient people. You had better study the difference between the voice that can beckon the spirit and the voice that can not beckon the spirit. You had better study the difference between the voice which careless or proud people utter and the voice which careful or alert people utter.

Furthermore, you had better listen to many various ethnic music and foreign languages. You had better be able to see the colors of ethnic music and of foreign languages and notice the smells, touch's senses, temperature of ethnic music and of foreign languages. You had better be able to classify the energies of voices and of sounds into the feeling of spring, the feeling of summer, the feeling of autumn and the feeling of winter. You had better be able to find what type of the spirit, of a devil and of an angel these ethnic music and foreign languages are apt to beckon. You had better imagine the fates, prosperity and tragedy that the feelings of these ethnic music and of foreign languages have brought about to the races that have sung such ethnic music and spoken in such languages.

When you can catch the energy of voice or of sound as if it were a substance, you can enter into another world and the universe through the energy of voice or of sound. For example, innumerable places of the universe have been exploding as if the universe beaten innumerable bass drums. If you can listen to a roll of the universe's drums, you will waver at the beginning and be able to temper yourself by its shock as if you were an iron. Its shock seems to deprive you of weakness, vagueness, timidity and indecision. Its shock can make you strengthen to become happy-healthy-efficient.

In this respect, I recommend that you had better read New Testament many times and catch the feeling of Christ and of Paul who did not fear the death and devoted themselves to the spirit. Christ was young, walked enough everyday and never made love (?), so he was very energetic and comported himself with confidence. Most of us can not imitate him because most of us have neither walked enough everyday nor saved sex energy at all. I think Christ could beckon the spirit easily and handle it freely. Christ could shoot out his strong immaterial fiber or third attention to an object, judge it accurately, control it, concentrate on it, and attain happy lucky feeling, inspiration, health and supernatural power through the success of concentration, too. So, he could do many marvelous acts. I feel the energy body (the consciousness) of Christ has been living in the universe and watching human-race.

I visited Jerusalem about 20 years ago. I felt as if I came back to my hometown when our bus was approaching Jerusalem just before sunset. I felt relieved and relaxed. My abdomen became warm. When I remembered the stone recently where Christ sat down all night at the last night on the earth, I saw that strong black energy suddenly overflowed into all over the world from this stone and the inner space turned to be red. I saw the inside of the Scriptures was burning, too. I can have understood that Christ said "I have come to set fire to the earth ". I can believe that Christ said "I will come and stay where a few men gather in my name".

If we read about Christ many times and imagine as if we were Christ in Israel 2000 years ago walking enough everyday and saving our sex energy as possible, our assemblage points (the core of consciousness) will easily move into the same interior of our physical bodies as that of Christ so that we can do the same acts as those of Christ did.

You will surely be able to meet the spirit sooner or later if you read the pages of meeting the spirit and imagine it as lively as possible.

We involving me are apt to be egotistic. We can not have forgotten personal indebtedness which other people have incurred to us, but have easily forgotten personal indebtedness which we have incurred to other people. In addition, to square certain personal indebtedness, I imagined good points of all women lively this early morning to whom I have incurred certain personal indebtedness in the course of my life. At the beginning of doing so following the way of "Saying Thank You" in the book-The Active Side of Infinity, I felt as if I opened up an old wound or took a bath of dirty hot water. But, today, I can feel the energy of my sex organ has become stronger and my awareness has become keener than yesterday. I can feel as if I unburdened a certain burden. I can feel happier and more airy. I think we have been badly influenced by the vindictive energy bodies of opposite sexes unconsciously as long as we have neither atoned nor appeased them.

Black energy parts from other energy and substance, and condenses. After condensation, some of black energy rushes to where it wants to approach. Black energy duplicates condensation and shooting each other. Black energy makes bones in physical body of human being. Black energy forms the shape of other energy or of substance and binds it together. I think transparent energy helps black energy because it invades into black energy and engulfs it .If all black energy and all transparent energy part from other energy or substance, other energy or substance will be exploded to pieces or melted.

Yellow energy is connected with some element of sugar. If yellow energy resolves and devours the black energy in other energy or sub-stance, other energy or substance will be exploded to pieces or melted. I think black energy is the core of our lives. If a machine is invented which can resolve and devour the black energy, it will be used as a weapon or medical treatment.

Furthermore, black energy within our bodies teaches us an accurate information as a silent voice when some of black energy within our bodies rushes from our physical bodies to where it wants to approach. I think we can feel most satisfied and happiest when some of our black energy within our bodies can rush to where it wants to approach.

Whenever I remember the events of my life in detail, I can recognize that I seldom can have shot out my immaterial fiber or third attention to an object from my body. As a result, I seldom can have succeeded in concentrating on it so that I seldom can have judged an outside object accurately, seldom can have controlled it, and seldom can have realized what I have imagined or planned. To my great regret, I am compelled to recognize that I have been stupid and a blockhead for long years. I have been so stubborn that I have almost ignored the spirit and my body-response. I have been apt to indulge in bad self-importance, undependable trust, hate and self-pity that have weakened me for long years.

I have often dealt with other people vaguely, too. I have often been irresponsible for a result. In such a case, my immaterial fiber or third attention is not used and is confined to my body. Such a vague behavior has weakened my immaterial fiber or third attention. As a result, I can not have shot out my immaterial fiber or third attention to other people from my body and have to have forgotten how to concentrate on other people and how to control other people.

I can not persuade or cure other people unless something like a rope of energy, a smoke or a fog flows to the bodies of other people from my body and invades the bodies of other people. A rope of energy, a smoke or a fog can neither flows to the bodies of other people from my body nor invades the bodies of other people whenever I eat too much, smoke, cut doing some proper body-exercise, constipate, remember unhappy-unhealthy-inefficient people, point the same aspect for long hours, ignore my comfortable body-response, make an unpleasant love with some female, complain, hate, get stuck or depressed, stay at powerless-spot for long hours or do not walk enough. Then, I can not persuade or cure other people.

Furthermore, I am surprised to find that I have almost made friends or acquaintances with the same people as me.

When most big men, founders, pioneers or enterprisers reach the pinnacle of success, they have begun to be unable to handle their immaterial fibers or third attention so that they have begun to be unable to concentrate on something, begun to go out the fire within their bodies, begun to have much stickiness of their bodies and begun to have bad complexion. Then, they have begun to have bad self-importance, undependable trust and self-pity, too. Most of them have ruined 3-10 later since they had become proud or careless.

Foolishly, I had smoked 2 packs of tobacco everyday until 5 years ago. The smoke of tobacco affected my head. If you read as many times as possible what I have written and remember your life lively at least 100 times, you will surely recognize that you have been almost stupid for long years, too.

For long years, I have aimlessly got angry at environmental pollution such as dirty air, water, river and sea, and at tree's having been cut down indiscriminately. I have indulged in such an aimless anger for long year. When you indulge in an aimless anger for long time, your immaterial fiber or third attention is not used and confined to your body so that it will easily become almost dead. If you get angry, you have to improve your surroundings by using your immaterial fiber or third attention. If you can not do so, you have to try to stop getting angry or have to try to run away or have to be indifferent by all means. Before you decide to fight (or how to fight) or run away or be indifferent, we have to be vague. But, you indulge in vagueness for long time, you will be rotten to the core.

In addition, I had hated several big vinyl houses in front of my house for about 20 years because the vegetables in these vinyl houses have the same feeling of melancholic. I could notice that I had indulged in a aimless anger and absorbed the same feeling of melancholic from these vegetables unconsciously for long years. A week ago when I walked beside these vinyl houses, I talked to the vegetables in these vinyl houses. By using my third attention, I said to these vegetables "Please, excuse human beings that will eat you soon. Don't get perverse as long as you live on the earth. Please, grow and live lively even though you can have short lives on the earth". When such a message could reach the vegetables in the vinyl house by me, beautiful transparent flash suddenly lightened in the vinyl house by me and the vegetables turned to be lively. Then, I could feel relieved and joyful.

Strangely, I can become relieved, relaxed, and can feel happier, healthier, more efficient whenever I can have recognized my stupidity and the bad influence of other people, of environmental pollution and of our surroundings deeply. The more we can recognize our stupidity deeply, the more we can have good health and supernatural power.

So, I recommend to you that you will remember your life in detail as many times as possible reading what I have written as many times as possible.

Now, I say thank you to the late Mr.Carlos Castaneda and the publishing companies that have published his books. Owing to his books, I can have proceeded more to a man of knowledge or a path of a warrior. When I read his last three books with the title-Magical Passes, The Wheel of Time and The Active Side of Infinity, I felt as if he knew that he would die of liver cancer in 1998. He seemed to have written before his death whatever he had been taught by don Juan Matus because he knew that he did not have the ability to become the successor to don Juan Matus. Mr. Carlos Castaneda hoped someone of those who read his books will become a successor to don Juan Matus.

According to some internet, he seemed to have earned about 20 million dollars to write his best seller books. I feel sorry that he died of liver cancer at the age of 72(?) in 1998. I wonder why he neither shot out his immaterial fiber or third attention to the energy body of don Genaro who is floating in the universe nor concentrated on it. Don

Genaro had loved and taught Mr. Carlos Castaneda very much before the departure to the universe. Don Genaro has much beautiful transparent green energy like light spring breeze that can cure liver disease easily. In addition, Mr. Carlos Castaneda might not have practiced what don Juan Matus taught him earnestly everyday.

But, I think Mr. Carlos Castaneda accomplished the feat to introduce the ancient Inca-knowledge (how to move our assemblage points freely, how to become healthy-happy-efficient, how to bring up our immaterial fibers or third attention, the hidden supernatural power of human being, how to beckon the spirit, how to become a psychic astronaut, and how to fuse with the universe without losing consciousness and live there for 2 billion years? as an inorganic being) to the world. He sent another new bible to the world.

"YOUTH"

Youth is not a time of life? it is a state of mind; it is a temper of the will, a quality of the imagination, a vigor of the emotions, a predominance of courage over timidity, of the appetite for adventure over love of ease.

Nobody grows old by merely living a number of years; people grow old only by deserting their ideals. Years wrinkle the skin, but to give up enthusiasm wrinkles the soul. Worry, doubt, self-distrust, fear and despair—these are the long, long years that bow the head and turn the growing spirit to back to dust.

Whether seventy or sixteen, there is in every being's heart the love of wonder, the sweet amazement at the stars and the starlike things and thoughts, the undaunted challenge of events, the unfailing childlike appetite for what next, and the joy and the game of life.

You are as young as your faith, as old as your doubt; as young as your self-confidence, as old as your fear, as young as your hope, as old as your despair.

So long as your heart receives messages of beauty, cheer, courage, grandeur and power from the earth, from man and from the Infinite, so long you are young.

When the wires are all down and all the central place of your heart is covered with the snows of pessimism and the ice of cynicism, then you are grown old indeed and may God have mercy on your soul.

By Ulman, an American poet

You can understand Ulman's poet, Youth completely because you have finished reading my book. Ulman's poet show us that we can erase the dirty stickiness which our complaints, the dirty energy body of other and devil have given to us, burn the beautiful strong fire within our bodies, shoot out our immaterial fibers or third attention to an outside object, judge it accurately, control it, succeed in concentrating on it, and attain happy lucky feeling, inspiration, health and supernatural power through the success of concentration. But, Mr. Ulman only shows us the phenomenon of peculiar happy lucky feeling, of inspiration, of health and of supernatural power, and has not shown how to beckon such a phenomenon. So, I have tried to show my readers how to beckon such a phenomenon as possible.

At first, to beckon the phenomenon of peculiar happy lucky feeling, of inspiration, of health and of supernatural power, you had better do some proper body-exercise everyday such as constricting anus 100 times in succession and denting navel 100 times in succession following the life style of long-lived British as possible patiently at least for 10 years. If you keep on doing so everyday, you will begin to burn the fire from within your body, burn out your dirty stickiness of your body and of your aura and release your immaterial fiber or third attention which has been confined to your dirty stickiness. As a result, you will able to learn to shoot out immaterial fiber or third attention to an outside object, judge it accurately, control it, succeed in concentrating on it, attain happy lucky feeling, inspiration, health and supernatural power through the success of concentration, realize what you imagine or plan, and follow your body-response little by little naturally.

It is very difficult that we keep on doing some proper body-exercise everyday following the life style of long-lived British as possible patiently at least for 10 years in spite of good fortune or misfortune. In most cases, if we become successful, we will become so careless or proud that we will stop doing some proper body-exercise everyday following the life style of long-lived British as possible patiently and ruin in 3-5 years or at the latest in 10 years. If we become unhappy-unhealthy-inefficient and fail in succession, we will have the sulks, stop doing so and ruin. I think it is the most important that you are modest or lively enough to keep on doing some proper body-exercise everyday following the life style of long-lived British as possible patiently at least for 10 years in spite of good fortune or misfortune.

If you keep on doing some proper body-exercise everyday such as constricting anus 100 times in succession and denting navel 100 times in succession following the life style of long-lived British as possible for a few months, you will begin to have good complexion and deprive your eyes of dreariness, irritation, hate, self-pity and irony. You will begin to be asked by many other people "You have changed. Has anything good happened to you recently?". If you keep on doing so for a year, you will begin to feel airy about your body or heart little by little. The views that you will look at will turn to be more beautiful and clearer than before. You may begin to hear purer sounds than before. Airy body and heart, more beautiful and clearer scenes and purer sounds will be able to heal the injury of your heart and encourage you.

Finally, I would like to express to earnest readers my deepest gratitude for finishing reading what I have written in bad English. The spirits bless you!

Furthermore, I say thank you to many spirits who have taught and guarded me in spite of my stupidity and stubbornness, many people who have shown me their kindness in my life and my wife.

## The End

# Bibliography

_A Separate Reality by Carlos Castaneda

_Enlightenment of Buddha (in Japanese) by Hiroyuki Nishigaki

_Executive ESP by Douglas Dean

_How to Attain Silent Knowledge (in Japanese) by Hiroyuki Nishigaki

_How to Concentrate on Your Breath and Stop it Automatically (in Japanese) by Hiroyuki Nishigaki

_Journey to Ixtlan by Carlos Castaneda

_Kabbala by Muriel. Doreal

_Keeper of Genesis by Robert Bauval and Graham Hancock

_LES PAGES IMMORTELLS DE NAPOLEON

_Magical Passes by Carlos Castaneda

_New Cosmos Series (in Japanese)

_Tales of Power by Carlos Castaneda

_Temper Your Body as Steel by Fan Ke Ping

_The Active Side of Infinity by Carlos Castaneda

_The Art of Dreaming by Carlos Castaneda

_The Eagle's Gift by Carlos Castaneda

_The Emerald-Tablets of Thoth-The-Atlantean by Muriel. Doreal

_The Fire from Within by Carlos Castaneda

_The Medicine of Ancient Chinese Yellow Emperor by Takeo Kosoto and Toshiyuki Hamada

_The Miracle of Mind Dynamics by Joseph Murphy

_The Original Sources of Buddha by Humio Mashutani (in Japanese)

_The Power of Silence by Carlos Castaneda

_The Revised English Bible(Oxford Cambridge)

_The Structure of The Earth by Youzou Hamano(in Japanese)

_The Second Ring of Power by Carlos Castaneda

_The Teachings of Don Juan by Carlos Castaneda

_The Wheel of Time by Carlos Castaneda

_Urban Shaman by Serge Kahili King

_Yoga Sutra by Turuzi Sahota (in Japanese)

_Rejuvenation and Unveiled Hidden Phenix by Hiroyuki Nishigaki

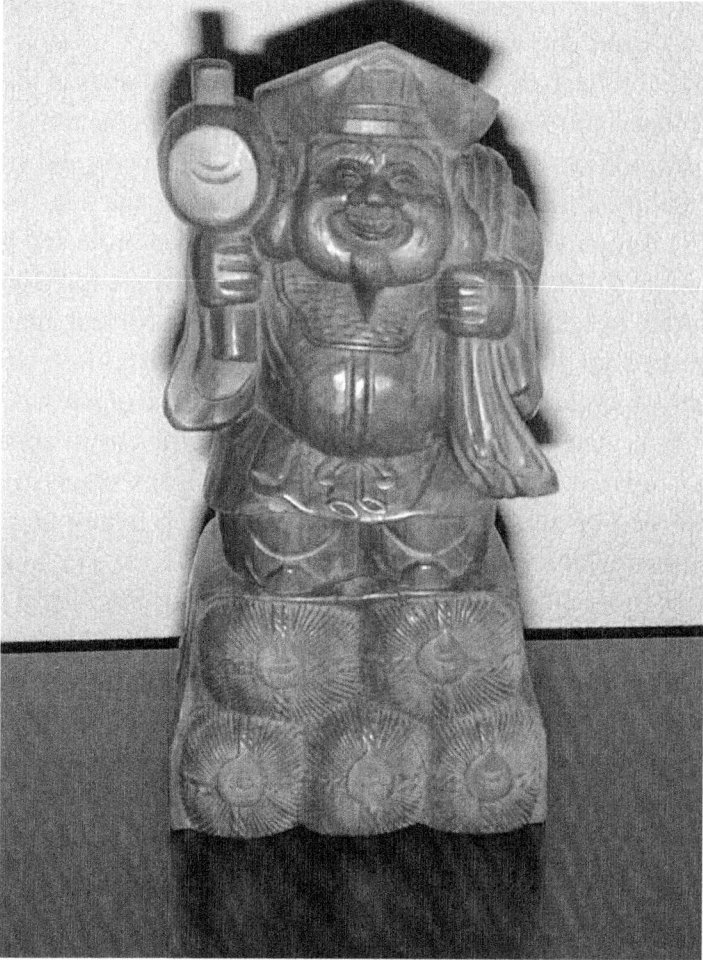

Mr. Nanboku Mizuno (1756–1834), the most famous Japanese man of physiognomy. He was out of a gangster. To study physiognomy, he worked for a barber, public bath and crematory. He studies as far as many sex organs and anuses.

He said (1) The part of a body between navel and anus is like a castle for a inner god where inner god lives (2) Happy-healthy-efficient men or women have well-developed waists, abdomens and buttocks. Happy-healthy-efficient men have strong kidneys and big tough sex organs (3) But, those who have too well- developed projected buttocks can not control their sexual desire or temper, so they are foolish and can not become a leader (4) Unhappy-unhealthy-inefficient man has a small, bridled-up, recurved-down, looked-right, looked-left, tapered or loose big sex organ. One who has such a male sex organ has a weak kidney (5) A man can become happy-healthy-efficient in spite of his small sex organ if he has a tough and hard small sex organ (6) A man with a bridled-up sex organ has cheerful makeup nature and is restlessly. A man with recurved-down sex organ is gloomy (7) A man who has a black glossy big sex organ and a well-developed gill will become a big man although he has a bridled-up sex organ (8) Happy-healthy-efficient female sex organ has a good complexion and good fragrance. It is buxom, heavy and moderately wet. It exists not at the front or back but at the center. It has beautiful well-developed clitoris and fin. The inside of her womb has a good complexion. Her womb has good constriction (9) Unhappy-unhealthy-inefficient female has a sex organ of bad complexion or a poor sex organ. It may exist at the front or back. Especially the color of her womb's inside is not beautiful. It may smell bad. She may have a big or small clitoris and fin of a bad complexion, too. Her sex organ may be dry or loose (10) Happy-healthy-efficient man or woman has a not-flabby, not-flaccid, not-nerveless anus which looks like the sun. Its radial lines looks like sun beams (11) Unhappy-unhealthy-inefficient man or woman has a weak kidney and few or thin hairs around a sex organ and an anus. Happy-healthy-efficient man or woman has a strong kidney and has many or thick hairs around a sex organ and an anus so that they can enjoy sex and have a rich heart.

Printed in Great Britain
by Amazon

81899229R00150